Scientific Tai Volume Two:

The Wu Jianquan Taijiquan Teachings of Chu Minyi

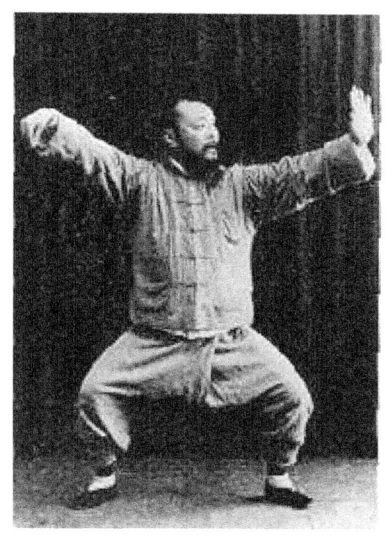

Translated by

Chen Faxing

Taijiquan Illustrated

Chu Minyi

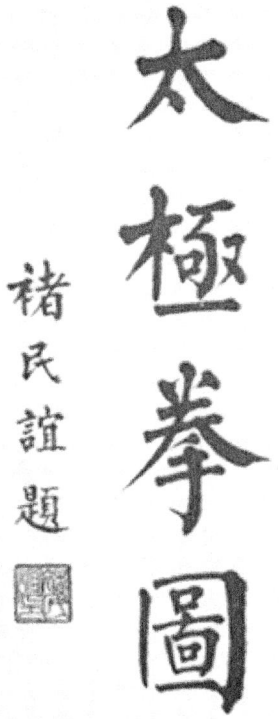

Taijiquan Illustrated

Inscribed by Chu Minyi

Translated by Chen Faxing

Title: Scientific Taijiquan Volume Two
Author: Chu Minyi
Translator: Chen Faxing
Publisher: Fa Xing Publishing
Year of Publication: 2023

Copyright © 2023 by Chen Faxing

All rights reserved. No part of this publication may be reproduced, distributed, or transmitted in any form or by any means, including photocopying, recording, or other electronic or mechanical methods, without the prior written permission of the publisher, except in the case of brief quotations embodied in critical reviews and certain other noncommercial uses permitted by copyright law.

Translator's Note:

The translation of this work was performed by Chen Faxing with the utmost care and attention to accuracy. However, any errors or discrepancies that may have occurred during the translation process are the sole responsibility of the translator.

Cover art designed by Chen Faxing.

Disclaimer:

The information and instructions presented in this book are intended for educational and instructional purposes only. The author and publisher have made every effort to ensure the accuracy and reliability of the content, but they do not assume any responsibility or liability for any errors, omissions, or consequences arising from the use of the information provided.

It is important to consult with a qualified instructor or practitioner before attempting any physical activities or exercises described in this book, particularly if you have any pre-existing medical conditions or concerns. The reader assumes all risks associated with the use of the information provided and agrees to release the author, translator, and publisher from any and all liability.

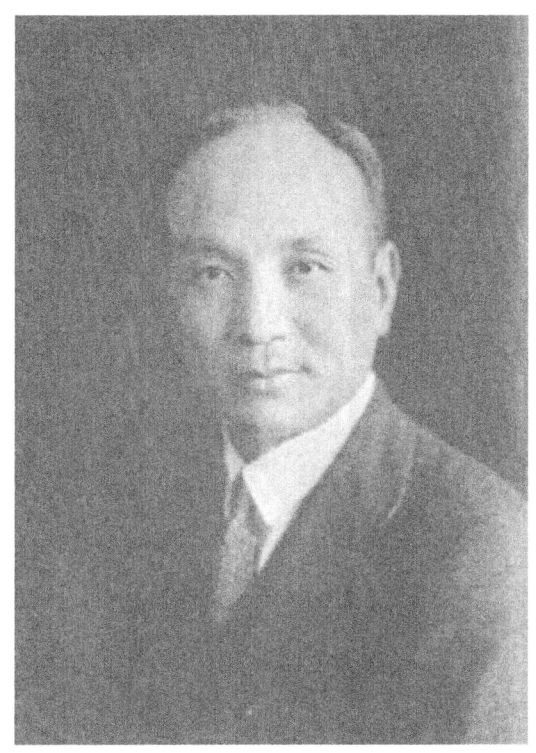

Photograph of Mr. Chu Minyi

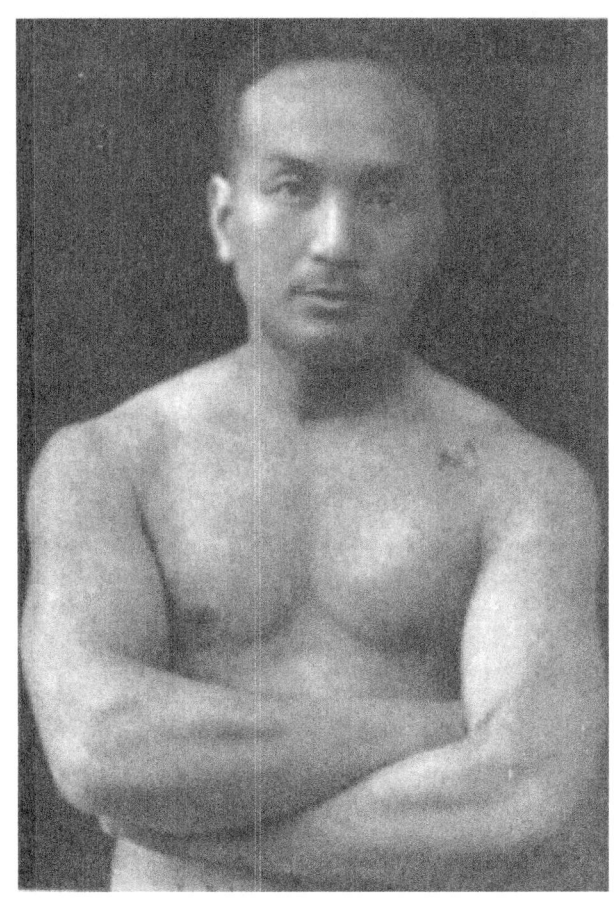

Physique of Mr. Chu Minyi

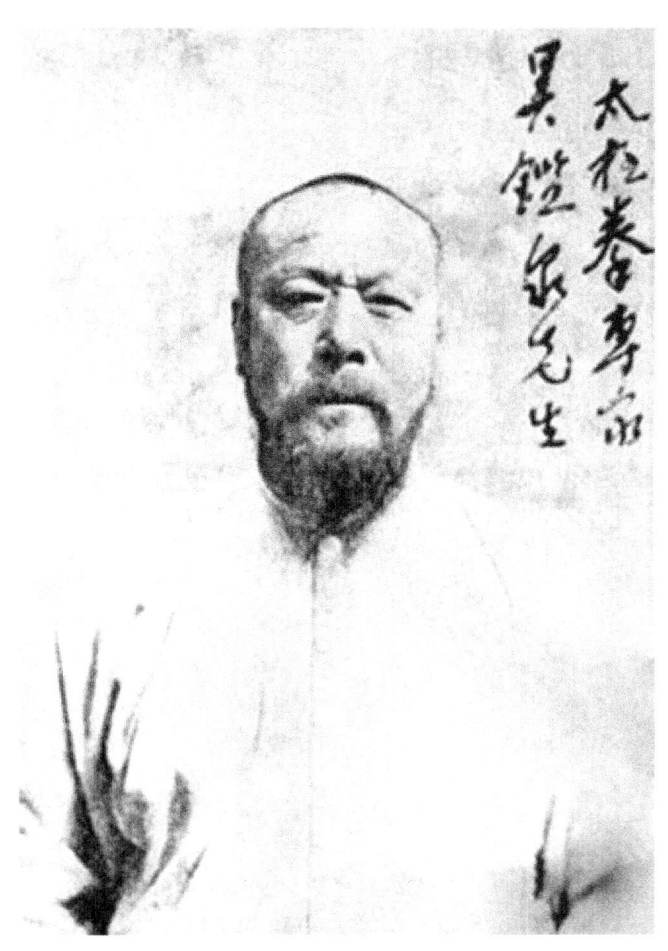

Photograph of Mr. Wu Jianquan

Mr. Wu Jianquan, Taijiquan expert

Short Biography of Chu Minyi

Chu Minyi, born in 1884 in the Wuxing district of Zhejiang province, China, was a prominent figure in the promotion of Chinese martial arts, particularly Taijiquan, to international audiences in the pre-World War II period. Despite his relatively brief involvement in the martial arts, Chu had a significant impact on shaping the global perception of these fighting systems.

Chu came from a gentry family, and his father, a distinguished physician, provided him with a solid education. He traveled to Japan in 1903 to study economics and politics, later moving to Singapore and France, where he joined a group of Chinese anarchists supporting revolutionary causes. He actively participated in the Tongmenghui, a revolutionary organization, and played a leadership role in Shanghai. However, disagreements led him to return to Europe, where he pursued degrees in medicine and pharmacology.

In 1925, following the death of Sun Yat Sen, Chu returned to China and settled in Guangzhou. He assumed positions in the Kuomintang (KMT) government, serving as Vice President of the Institut Franco-Chinois and later earning a doctorate from the University of Strasbourg. Additionally, he became the head of the medical school at Guangdong University.

Chu's passion for Taijiquan emerged during this period, and he described himself as a "Taiji addict." While he had not studied martial arts extensively during his time abroad, he became deeply involved in the practice upon returning to China. He received instruction from renowned Taijiquan teacher Wu Jianquan and later studied with other notable practitioners such as Wang Zhiqun, Wu Zizhen, and Xu Zhiyi.

Chu's interest in martial arts aligned with the efforts of the Kuomintang to establish a national martial arts program through the Central Guoshu Institute. He recognized the potential of martial arts to contribute to the strengthening of the nation and sought to modernize and "scientize" them. In an article published in 1928, Chu outlined his vision of promoting guoshu (national martial arts) and presenting them to the world, emphasizing the need to incorporate scientific methods, mechanics, psychology, physiology, and hygiene into martial arts research and practice.

Chu's endeavors in promoting the martial arts went beyond his personal practice. He published manuals on Wu style Taijiquan and introduced innovations of his own. He also wrote prefaces for other martial arts manuals, providing inscriptions and calligraphy. Through these activities, Chu sought to systematize and spread the martial arts, giving them scholarly and methodological credibility.

Chu's promotion of the martial arts was not only driven by a domestic agenda but also aimed to shape international perceptions of China. He recognized the strategic value of martial arts in public diplomacy, considering the success of Japan's cultivation of Budo as a means to project strength, uniqueness, and legitimacy. By showcasing the physical strength and spiritual will of the Chinese people, Chu hoped to gain Western support in resisting Japanese imperialist claims.

Although Chu's efforts to popularize the Chinese martial arts in the West prior to World War II did not achieve their intended goals, his work laid the foundation for future developments. His emphasis on modernization, scientific methods, and public diplomacy foreshadowed later initiatives to promote martial arts as a tool of statecraft. Chu's life remains a remarkable and tragic story, with further research needed to uncover additional details about his personal life and motivations.

Table of Contents

Huang Chuiju's Preface

Chu Minyi's Preface

(1) Theory of Taijiquan

(2) Taijiquan Classics

(3) Thirteen Postures Song

(4) Explanation of the Mental Aspects of the Thirteen Postures

(5) Push Hands Song

(6) Names and Sequence of Taijiquan Postures

Explanation of Taijiquan Push Hands and Equipment

Taijiquan Pole Illustrations

Taijiquan Ball Illustrations

Applications of Taijiquan Pole

Applications of Taijiquan Ball

Huang Chujiu's Preface

For a nation to exist permanently in the world without being eliminated by natural selection, it must possess a complete scientific civilization, a rigorous social organization, a spirit of evolution in every individual, and a robust physique. However, all scientific civilization, material civilization, and spiritual civilization rely on a strong physique for their cultivation and maintenance. Therefore, the essential condition for the survival of a nation is nothing other than a robust physique. In our Chinese civilization, which has lasted for five thousand years and has a population of four hundred million, its ability to nourish and reproduce until today without extinction is also nothing other than the fact that our ancestors and ancestors had a strong physique. In recent times, there has been an emphasis on culture over martial arts, resulting in the physical constitution of the people weakening. All scientific civilization and material civilization cannot be fully embraced and studied. As a result, the national wealth has become impoverished. Therefore, the decline of a country is invariably accompanied by poverty and weakness. It is not without reason. Today, the key to saving the country lies in alleviating poverty and weakness. Enhancing material civilization, producing domestic goods, and plugging the leaking vessel are one aspect of alleviating poverty. Together with hygiene and medicine, supplementing the physical strength of the people is another aspect of alleviating weakness. I founded Jiufu Company and released products like the Hundred-Year Machine Supplement Patch with the same purpose. However, apart from medication, there is also the path of martial arts to strengthen the body. Our country's martial arts have the earliest origins and can be regarded as outstanding in the world. That Eastern Peninsula, having obtained a fragment of our martial arts, strengthened its country through Bushido (the way of the warrior). We, on the other hand, abandoned and neglected it, resulting in accumulated weakness. Now, those with aspirations have come to realize the importance of martial arts and are loudly advocating for research, as well as personally practicing it. Mr. Chu Minyi, a member of the Central Committee, is particularly proficient in martial arts, considering Taijiquan as the essence of martial arts. Regardless of gender or age, anyone can practice it, and the magnitude of its effectiveness depends on the depth of the practitioner's attainment. It is advantageous and flawless, making it the most perfect. Therefore, it is vigorously promoted with utmost effort. Moreover, several apparatuses for practicing Taijiquan have been invented to elucidate its essence. When I heard about this, I admired it and wished to learn from it. Mr. Chu graciously showed me the Taijiquan pictures he took with Mr. Wu Jianquan. Mr. Wu Jianquan is a senior in the realm of Taijiquan with profound accomplishments. With his pictures, I can practice step by step. I dare not keep it to myself and intend to widely publish it for the benefit of the public. Mr. Chu generously agreed and provided explanations. Despite Mr. Chu's busy and important responsibilities for the country, he remains enthusiastic about this matter. This is worthy of respect. On the day of publication, I apologize for my lack of literary skill in writing this preface.

Written by Huang Chujiu at the Zhi Zu Lu in the spring of the 18th year of the Republic (1929).

Chu Minyi's Preface

The purpose of martial arts is to cultivate the body and mind and invigorate the spirit. However, the martial arts in our country have ancient origins, and due to the differences in postures and functions, they are categorized and named differently. Some emphasize the extraordinary and mysterious, while others value simplicity and accessibility. Not all of them have fully developed into physical education, and the divisions and disputes are endless. Tracing back to their origins, there are ultimately two major schools: Wudang and Shaolin. Wudang emphasizes softness and internal cultivation of strength, while Shaolin focuses on firmness and external display of strength. In recent times, the influence of Shaolin has grown significantly. As it spreads widely and the number of schools and styles increases, there is a tendency to pursue novelty and uniqueness, deviating from the essence of physical education. Beginners who learn it often put in double the effort for half the result, and it is particularly harmful to those with weak bodies. Therefore, I have chosen not to adopt it. Taijiquan, on the other hand, is the most accessible and effective martial art among the internal styles in developing physical education. I have developed a great fondness for it and practice it daily without interruption, regardless of the weather. The longer I practice, the more I realize its infinite subtleties. Its magnificent benefits and numerous merits are truly unparalleled by other martial arts. Here, I will describe its postures, movements, intentions, issuing of strength, agility, and health cultivation.

(1) Postures

The postures of Taijiquan are numerous, (see picture) totaling the Five Elements and the Eight Trigrams, known as the Thirteen Postures. What are the Five Elements? They are advancing, retreating, looking left, and looking right, and standing still.

What are the Eight Trigrams? They are warding off, rolling back, pressing, pushing, plucking, splitting, elbowing, and leaning. These thirteen postures are the essential path that Taijiquan practitioners must go through. By practicing them daily without interruption for several years, one's proficiency in the profoundness of the martial art will naturally unfold, bringing significant benefits.

(2) Movements

The movements of Taijiquan should be slow and even. Unlike external martial arts that may appear fast and effective, they often carry inherent flaws. Taijiquan, however, focuses on the activation of tendons and bones. Therefore, all movements should be performed with softness and harmony. Only through slowness can one achieve softness, and only through evenness can one achieve harmony. All movements are circular in shape, and within each circle, changes between emptiness and fullness occur. The infinite subtleties lie in these changes between emptiness and fullness. Beginners may not fully comprehend this, but with prolonged practice, they will develop a natural familiarity and endless enjoyment. It not only stretches and relaxes the tendons and bones but also harmonizes the blood and qi, making it an ideal method for developing physical education while simultaneously cultivating the mind.

(3) Intentions

When practicing Taijiquan, one should rely solely on naturalness, not on exerting force or qi but on using intention. Using excessive force results in clumsiness, and using excessive qi leads to stagnation. Therefore, sinking the qi and relaxing the force are crucial. When the qi sinks, the inhalation and exhalation become harmonious, and when the force relaxes, the innate force is activated while eliminating the extraneous force. Innate force is the inherent strength, while extraneous force is the forced strength. The former flows smoothly, while the latter resists. Taijiquan emphasizes accepting the opponent's force and countering with softness, thus requiring no excessive force. In contrast, external martial arts often rely on forced exertion, making it challenging for even the strong to achieve. Improper practice of such forceful methods leads to inherent flaws. Those who persist in forceful methods exhaust their strength without subtlety. Despite years of practice, their external strength may seem to improve superficially, but internally, their power remains unchanged. In Taijiquan, although excessive force and qi are not used, the focus of practice lies entirely in one's intention. By utilizing intention, the internal strength is stored, not revealed externally; the qi sinks to the dantian, not stagnating in the chest. Without excessive force or qi, through long-term practice, the accumulation of internal energy and strength grows. When necessary, it can be freely applied without difficulty or forced exertion. It is similar to laborers who work all day, utilizing their strength and qi. However, their energy is completely expended without accumulation. Therefore, even after years of labor, their strength and qi remain the same. The same applies to the forceful methods of external martial arts.

(4) Issuing Power

There is a distinction between strong and soft power: What is strong power? Regardless of the magnitude, it contains resistance and an unstoppable force. That is called strong power. What is soft power? It extends and contracts with the opponent's power without resistance. That is called soft power. The brilliance of Taijiquan lies in its ability to accept the opponent's power without immediately launching an offensive. Instead, it uses its sticking and yielding power to neutralize the opponent's stubborn force. When the opponent's strike fails, and they intend to launch another attack, then Taijiquan seizes the opportunity, follows their movement, and turns defense into offense. As a result, when the opponent is exhausted and their balance is disrupted, rarely do they succeed. The movements of Taijiquan do not consist of countless circular forms, but within the circular form, the center of gravity is constantly established with rooted feet. Even if the opponent's power is strong, it is redirected using the method of accepting and countering. Once the opponent's force is exerted and their balance is lost, Taijiquan takes control. This is known as evading the real and striking the empty, utilizing softness to overcome hardness.

(5) Agility

As the saying goes, practice makes perfect. Taijiquan embodies this idea and those who engage in it deeply understand its essence. The refinement of Taijiquan depends on the depth of one's practice. With deep practice, one gains a thorough understanding of the changes between emptiness and fullness. Once these changes are understood, one can seek out the path of ingenuity within them. The power used in Taijiquan is light, agile, and rounded. It differs greatly from the focused and rigid power used in external martial arts. Also, because excessive force and qi are not used, it can be sustained without depletion. The movements are circular, providing stability to the center of gravity at all times. A stable center of gravity leads to a solid foundation, free from the invasion of external forces.

(6) Health Preservation

Martial arts are originally a form of physical education, with health preservation as the primary goal. However, this is not the case with forceful methods of external martial arts. Only Taijiquan truly excels at health preservation and can be practiced by people of all strengths, ages, and conditions. The development of our bodies should aim for balance, following a certain physiological process. Intense exercises that deviate from this process often yield negative results. The movements of

Taijiquan are gentle and exceptional, engaging the entire body in each movement without bias towards any specific part. Furthermore, due to the gentle and agile nature of the movements, it can harmonize qi and blood, cultivate one's disposition, and adhere to the physiological process for balanced development. During practice, there is no need to exert excessive force or qi, making it accessible even for the elderly, weak, or those with illnesses. The saying "recovery from illness and longevity" is indeed not an empty claim.

In the 14th year of my life, I traveled from Guangdong to Beiping, where I had the opportunity to visit Mr. Wu Jianquan, a renowned master of Taijiquan. Mr. Wu was a true inheritor of the authentic Wudang lineage of Taijiquan. At that time, I requested him to demonstrate various postures of Taijiquan, which I captured in photographs for further study and observation. Upon returning to Guangdong, I, along with Wang Zhiqun and Wu Zizhen, dedicated our evenings to researching and seeking progress. When I arrived in Shanghai, I met Mr. Xu Zhijun, and we engaged in discussions about Taijiquan. Mr. Xu had profound knowledge and extensive research on the principles of Taijiquan. He had previously published a book titled "A Brief Discussion on Taijiquan," which became widely known. He was a distinguished disciple of Mr. Wu Jianquan. Now that Mr. Wu has also come to Shanghai, I have the opportunity to continue learning from him. Notably, Taijiquan experts such as the Yang family, Shao Hou, and Chengfu reside in the capital. Additionally, Chengfu's accomplished disciple, Mr. Chen Weiming, is also in Shanghai. With the collective efforts of these Taijiquan practitioners, our path can be considered promising in terms of advancing and developing Taijiquan. Therefore, Jiufu Company entrusted me to create a film to be produced as a picture booklet, aiming to widely disseminate Taijiquan. I, too, highly value this martial art and strive to promote its worth. Hence, I cannot deny their request, and despite my limited ability, I will do my best to explain its functions and highlight its advantages within these simple pages.

Chu Minyi of Wuxing, Wuzhou February 5th, 1929 Written at the Shanghai Sino-French Industrial Specialized School

(1) Theory of Taijiquan

In every movement, the entire body must be light and agile, interconnected and harmonized. The qi should be expansive, while the spirit should be internally focused, without any deficiencies, protrusions, or interruptions. The root is in the feet, manifested through the legs, controlled by the waist, and expressed through the fingertips. From the feet to the legs to the waist, there must be a complete unity of qi. Only by moving forward or retreating can one seize opportunities and advantageous positions. Any failure to seize opportunities and positions will result in a scattered and disordered body, and the remedy lies in the legs and waist. This principle applies to all directions: up, down, forward, backward, left, and right. All of this is the intention, not external appearance. Up corresponds to down, forward corresponds to backward, and left corresponds to right. If the intention is to lift an object and then crush it, the root will be severed, causing swift and undeniable damage. Clear distinctions between empty and full should be made. Each place has its own emptiness and fullness, yet overall, every place contains this concept of emptiness and fullness. The entire body should be connected without the slightest interruption.

Long Fist is like the vastness of the Yangtze River and the sea, flowing endlessly. The Thirteen Techniques consist of Peng, Lu, Ji, An, Cai, Lie, Zhou, Kao, representing the Eight Trigrams. Advance, retreat, look left, gaze right, and maintain the center represent the Five Elements. Peng, Lu, Ji, An correspond to Qian, Kun, Kan, Li, the four cardinal directions. Cai, Lie, Zhou, Kao correspond to Xun, Zhen, Dui, Gen, the four diagonal directions. Advance, retreat, look left, gaze right, and maintain the center correspond to Metal, Wood, Water, Fire, and Earth, respectively. (Note: It is said that this is the discourse left behind by the venerable Zhang Sanfeng of Wudang Mountain, not merely a skill or technique for the sake of longevity and health for heroes throughout the world.)

(2) Taijiquan Classic

Taijiquan is born from the ultimate limit, the mechanism of movement and stillness, the mother of yin and yang. When in motion, it separates; when still, it integrates. There is no excess or deficiency. It follows curves and extends with them. When the opponent is forceful, I am yielding, which is called "zou." When I am compliant and follow the opponent's back, it is called "nian." If the opponent moves swiftly, I respond swiftly; if the opponent moves slowly, I follow slowly. Although there are countless variations, the underlying principle remains consistent. Through practice and gradual understanding of jin, one attains spiritual enlightenment. However, without persistent effort, one cannot suddenly comprehend it. The crown of the head is empty, with the energy sinking to the dantian, maintaining perfect balance. It appears and disappears unpredictably. When the left side is heavy, the left side becomes empty; when the right side is heavy, the right side becomes empty. When tilting upward, it becomes increasingly high; when leaning downward, it becomes increasingly deep. Advancing makes it longer; retreating makes it shorter. Even a feather cannot be added, and a fly cannot land. People do not perceive me, but I alone perceive others. Heroes become invincible due to this. There are numerous peripheral styles, although they may have distinguishing characteristics, they all boil down to the principles of strength overcoming weakness and slowness yielding to speed. The ability to strike forcefully when strong, and to yield when slow, is an innate natural capability. It has nothing to do with acquired skills. Observing the phrase "four ounces deflects a thousand pounds," it is evident that it is not about overpowering with strength. Observing how the elderly can fend off a crowd, speed alone is not the determining factor. To stand like a balanced scale, to move like a spinning wheel, to sink when pressed, to be stagnant when double-weighted—these are the results of years of dedicated training. Those who cannot transform their practice after many years are usually hindered by their own limitations. The affliction of being double-weighted remains unrecognized. To avoid this ailment, one must understand the principles of yin and yang. Sticking is synonymous with "zou," and "zou" is synonymous with sticking. Yin cannot separate from yang, and yang cannot separate from yin. When yin and yang complement each other, one truly understands jin. After comprehending jin, the more you practice, the more refined it becomes. Silent understanding and contemplation gradually lead to achieving what the heart desires. It is fundamentally about abandoning oneself to follow others. Many make the mistake of discarding what is close at hand and seeking what is far away. This is akin to missing by a hair but deviating by a thousand miles. As a learner, one must not neglect careful discernment.

(3) Thirteen Postures Song

In the realm of movement, the thirteen forms reside,

Never underestimate their power, don't let them slide.

Their essence springs forth from the waist's hidden seam,

Embrace the interplay of real and unreal, it's no idle dream.

Let the qi flow freely, unimpeded in its course,

In stillness, a touch of motion, an unyielding force.

Adapt to the changes, display your wondrous skill,

With focused intent, every movement you fulfill.

Effortlessly, the mind holds each form in its grasp,

Unaware of the toil, no struggle in this clasp.

In the depths of your waist, attention must reside,

A relaxed belly, soaring qi, to the crown it'll glide.

Balanced and light, the body poised with grace,

As if floating, every step finds its rightful place.

To enter this path, guidance must be bestowed,

Endless dedication, the practice steadily flowed.

If you ask, what criteria should one employ,

Between intent and qi, a harmony to enjoy.

The mind and qi reign, bones and flesh obey,

Seeking longevity, embracing life's precious ray.

Sing, oh sing, this song of a hundred and forty lines,

Each word sincere, revealing truth that brightly shines.

Without delving into this wisdom's sacred core,

Fruitless would be the effort, regret forevermore.

(4) Explanation of the Mental Aspects of the Thirteen Postures

To cultivate the art of Taijiquan, one must learn to move with the heart leading the breath, aiming for a state of deep composure. This allows for the gathering and consolidation of energy, permeating even the bones themselves. By harnessing the power of qi, one can achieve fluidity and ease in the body's movements.

Elevating the spirit is crucial, as it prevents sluggishness and excessive heaviness. It is said to be akin to having one's head suspended from above. The combination of intention (xin) and vital energy (qi) must be flexible and responsive, allowing for seamless transitions between real and illusory movements.

When initiating motion, it is important to maintain a sense of calmness and relaxed alertness, focusing on a singular direction. Meanwhile, the body should stand upright with a centered and balanced posture, acting as a support from all sides.

The circulation of qi should resemble a string of nine pearls, flowing effortlessly throughout the body, bringing benefits in every direction. This agile movement is akin to the strength and resilience of finely crafted steel. The form should be reminiscent of a falcon pouncing on its prey, and the spirit should mirror that of a cat capturing a mouse.

In stillness, one should embody the unwavering presence of a mountain, while in motion, flow like the currents of a river. The accumulation of strength should resemble drawing a bow, and the release of force should mirror the swift release of an arrow. Seeking straightness within the curved movements, one should aim to connect and maintain continuity.

Advance and retreat should be accomplished through seamless transitions, and flexibility should be cultivated to the utmost degree. Softness and pliancy are the foundation for hardness and strength. Only by mastering the art of breathing can one truly achieve a state of fluidity and agility. Qi should be nurtured with directness and harmlessness, while strength should be accumulated with curved and coiled movements.

The mind serves as the commander, while the qi acts as the flagbearer, and the waist functions as the standard-bearer. The pursuit begins with expanding and opening up, followed by contracting and consolidating. Only through these efforts can one attain a level of meticulous refinement in their practice.

(5) Push Hands Song

In Taijiquan, it is crucial to perform ward-off, rollback, press, and push with sincerity. The upper and lower body should follow each other, making it difficult for the opponent to advance. Let them exert their mighty force against me, as I utilize the principle of "four ounces deflecting a thousand pounds." I draw them in, causing their attack to miss, and then respond with a seamless combination.

Furthermore, it is said, "If the opponent doesn't move, I don't move. If the opponent makes a slight move, I move first." The power appears relaxed yet not relaxed, ready to expand yet not fully expanded. The power breaks, but the intention remains unbroken.

(6) Names and Sequence of Taijiquan Postures

(1) Taijiquan (Picture 1)

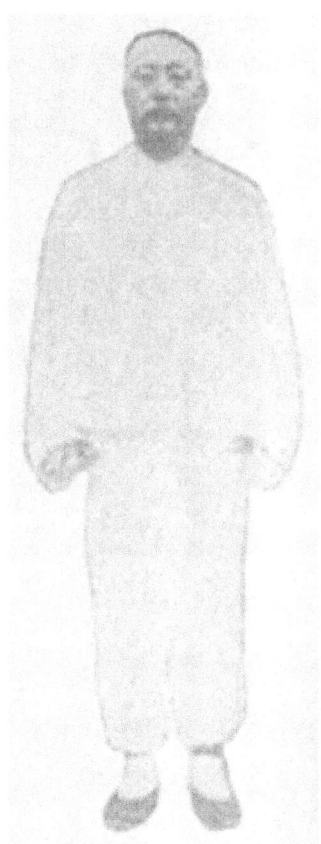

(2) Taijiquan Starting Form (Picture 2)

(3) Grasp the Sparrow's Tail 1 (Picture 3)

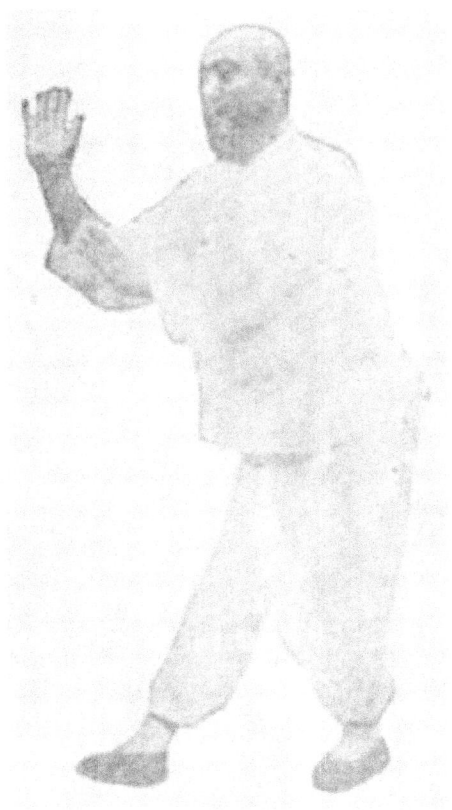

(4) Grasp the Sparrow's Tail 2 (Picture 4)

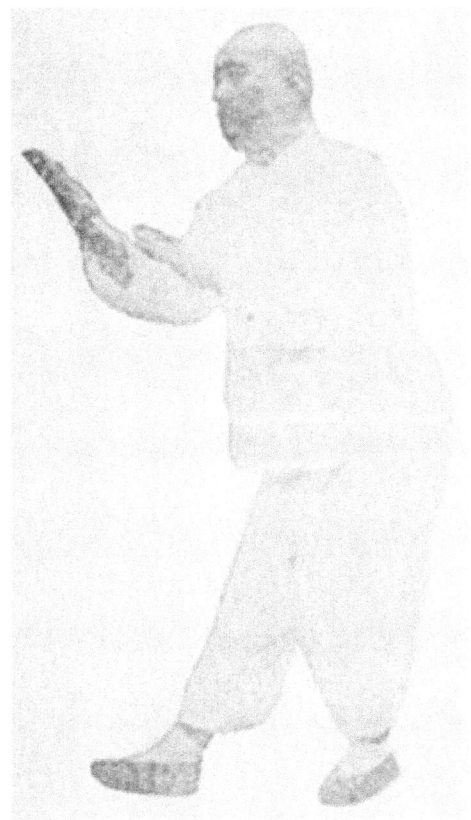

(5) Grasp the Sparrow's Tail 3 (Picture 5)

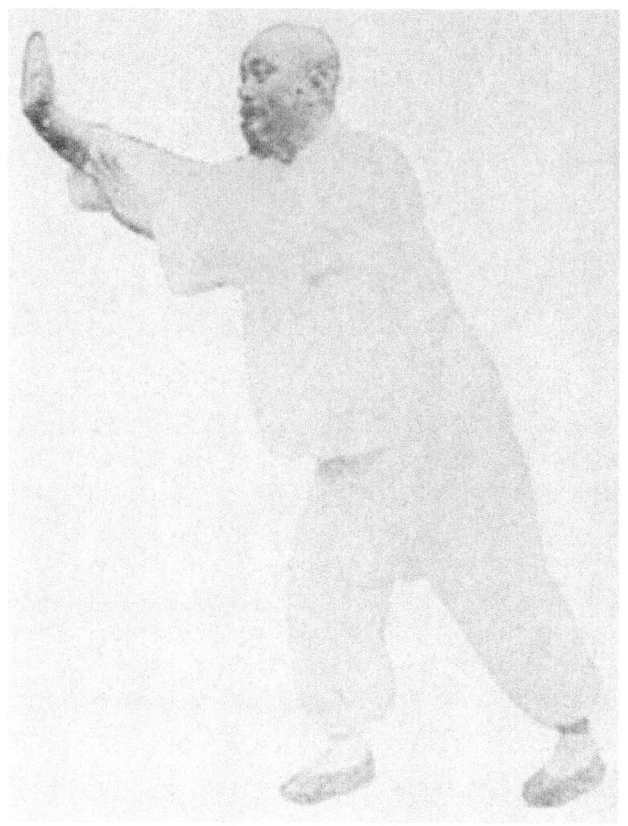

(6) Single Whip (Picture 6)

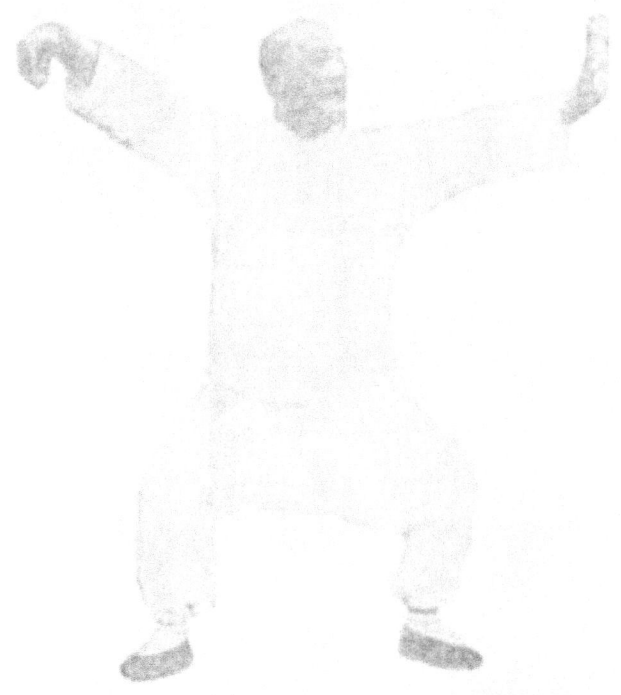

(7) Raise Hands, First Posture (Picture 7)

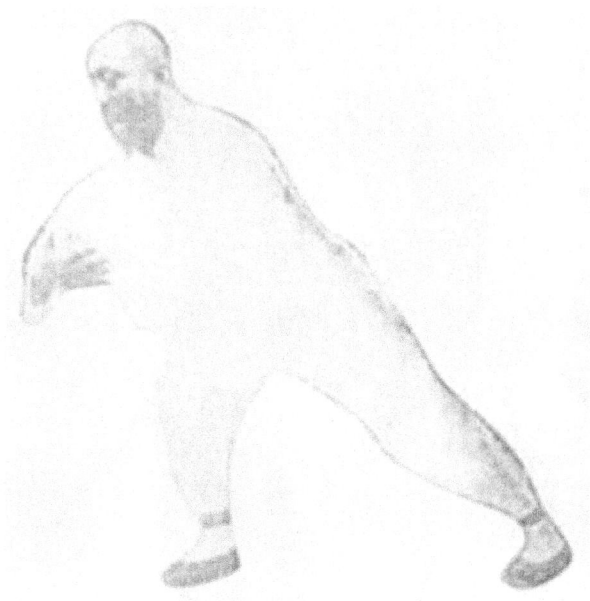

(8) Raise Hands, Second Posture (Picture 8)

(9) White Crane Spreads Its Wings, First Posture (Picture 9)

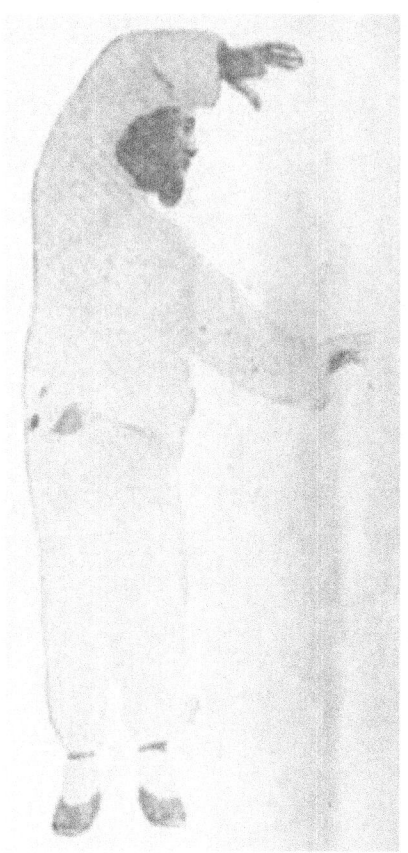

(10) White Crane Spreads Its Wings, Second Posture (Picture 10)

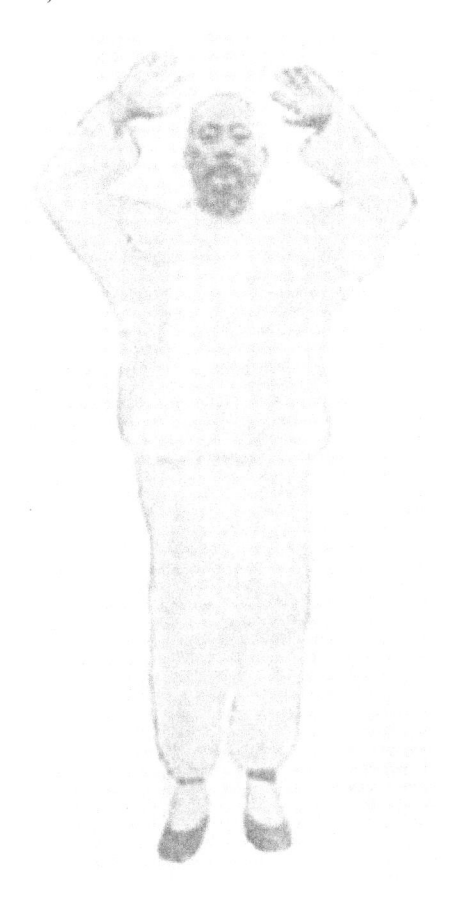

(11) Brush Knee and Twist Step (Left) (Picture 11)

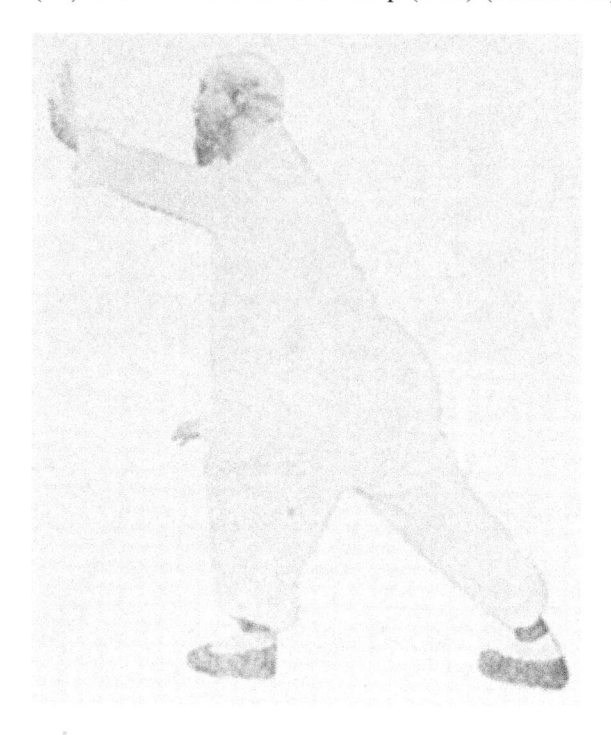

(12) Brush Knee and Twist Step (Right) (Picture 12)

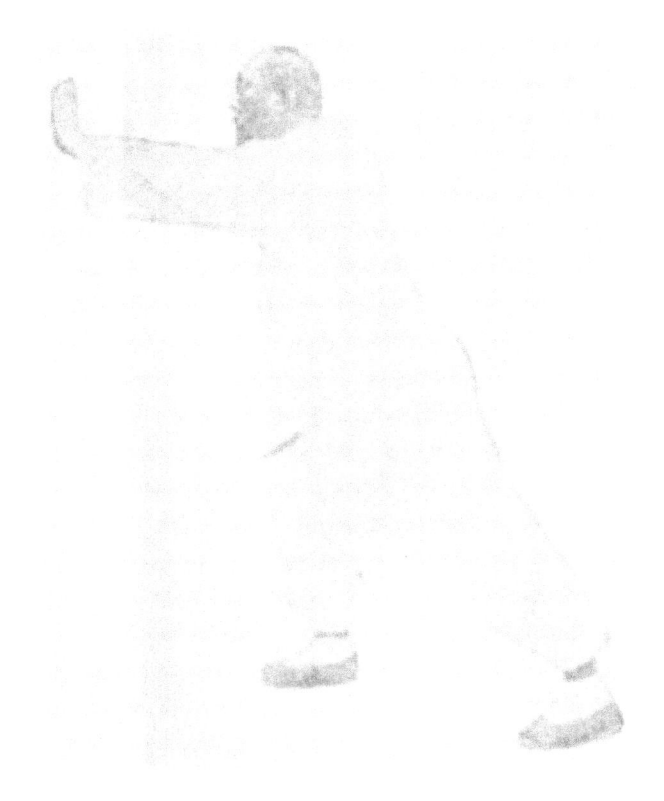

(13) Play the Pipa (Picture 13)

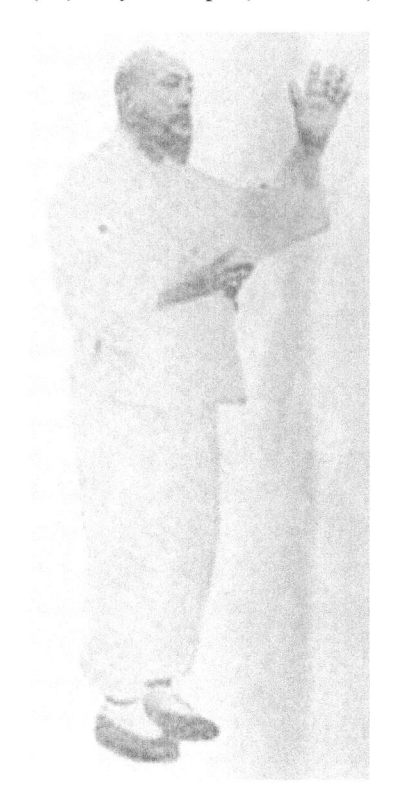

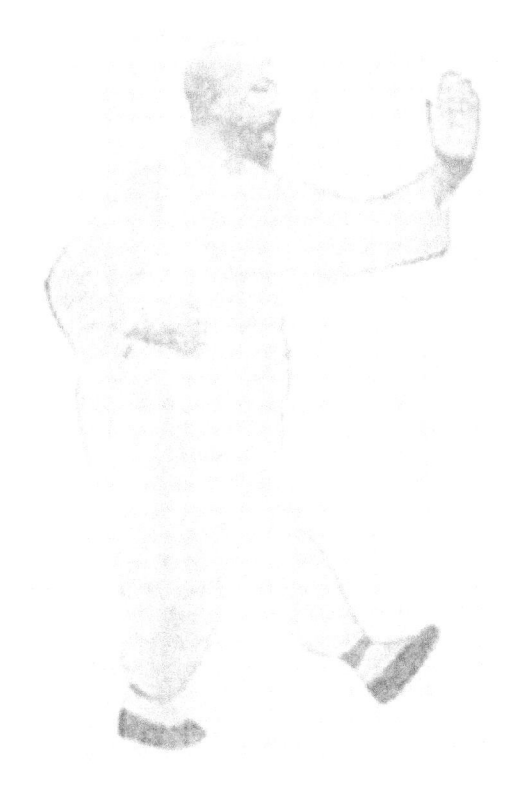

(14) Step Forward, Deflect, Parry, and Punch (Picture 14)

(15) Step Forward, Deflect, Parry, and Punch (Picture 15)

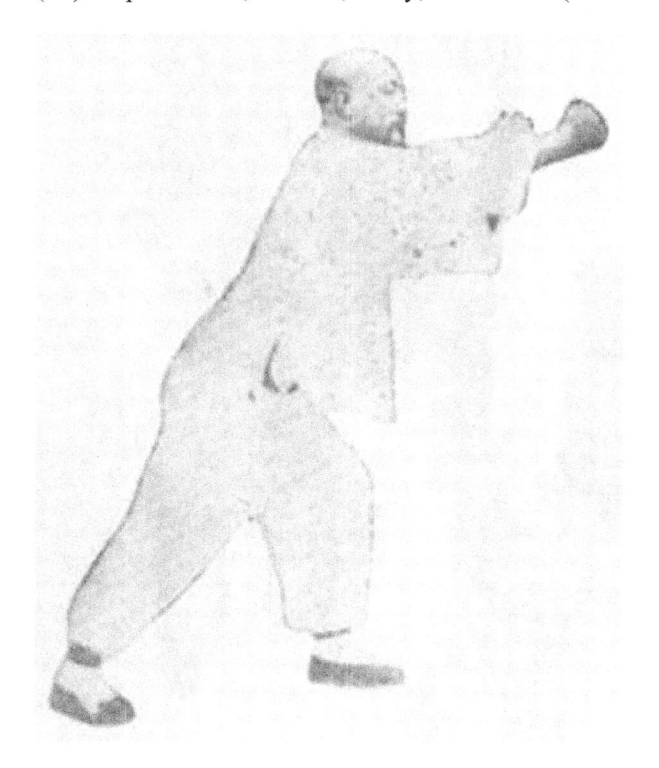

(16) Closing and Sealing (Picture 16)

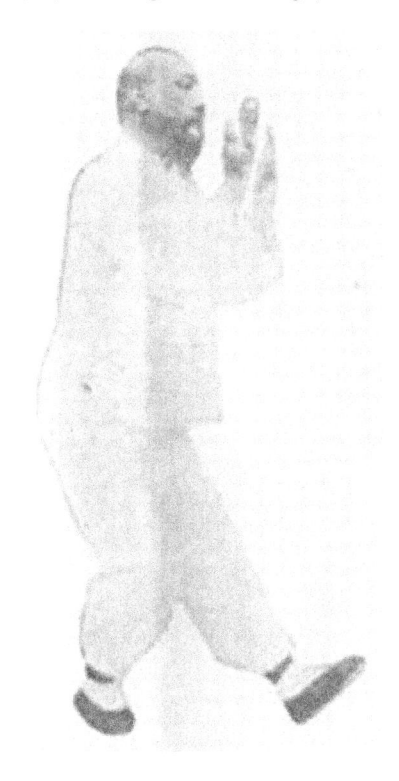

(17) Embrace the Tiger and Return to Mountain (Pictures 17a and 17b)

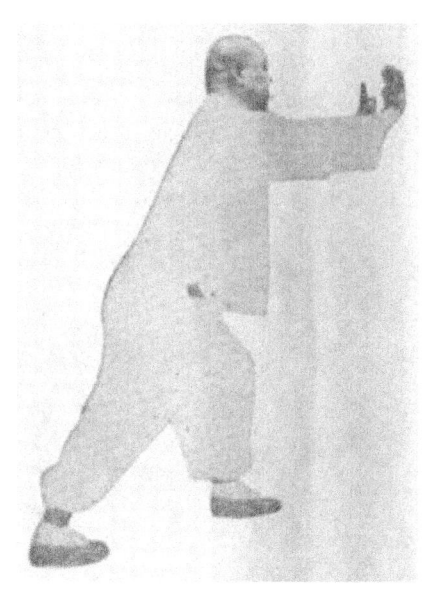

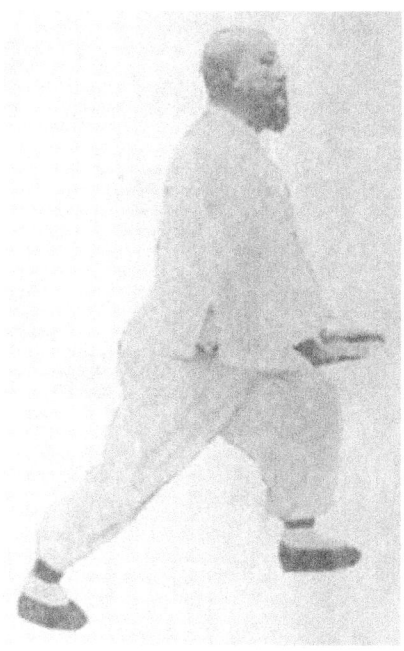

(18) Grasping the Knee and Twisting Step (Picture 11)

(19) Grasp the Sparrow's Tail (Picture 3)

(20) Diagonal Single Whip (Picture 18)

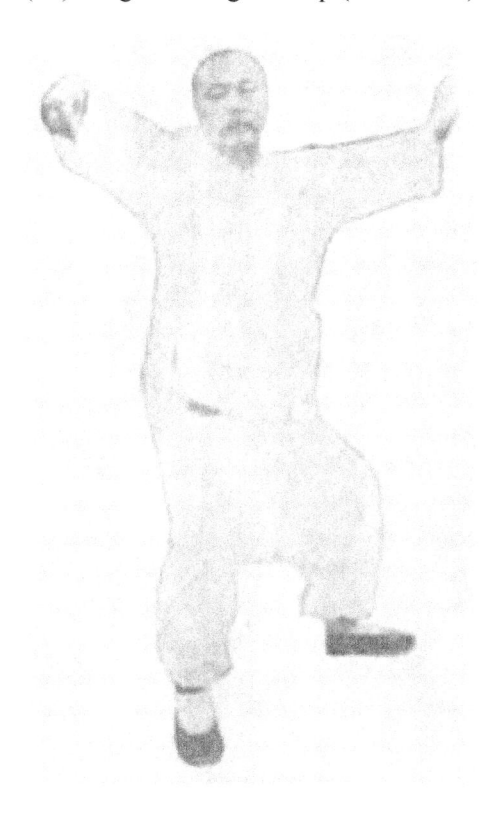

(21) Punch Under Elbow (Picture 19)

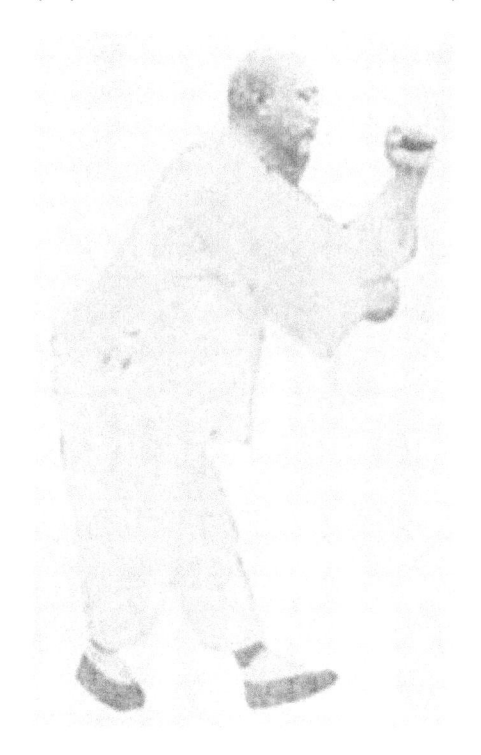

(22) Retreat and Repulse Monkey 1 (Picture 20)

(23) Retreat and Repulse Monkey 2 (Picture 21)

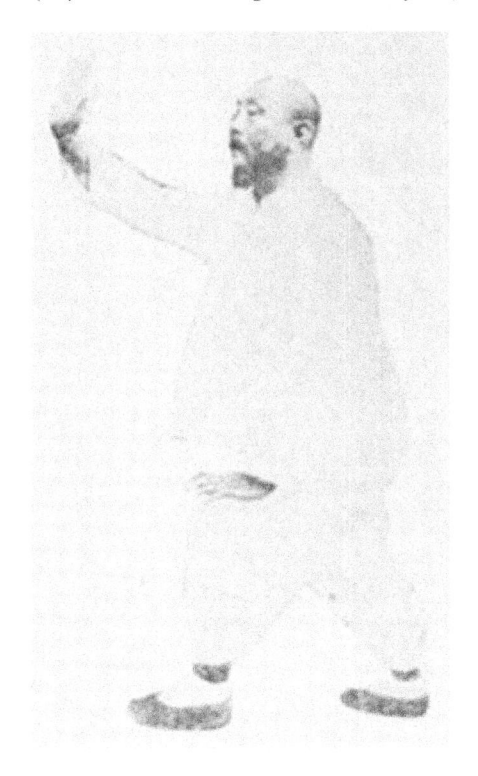

(24) Slant Flying Posture (Picture 22)

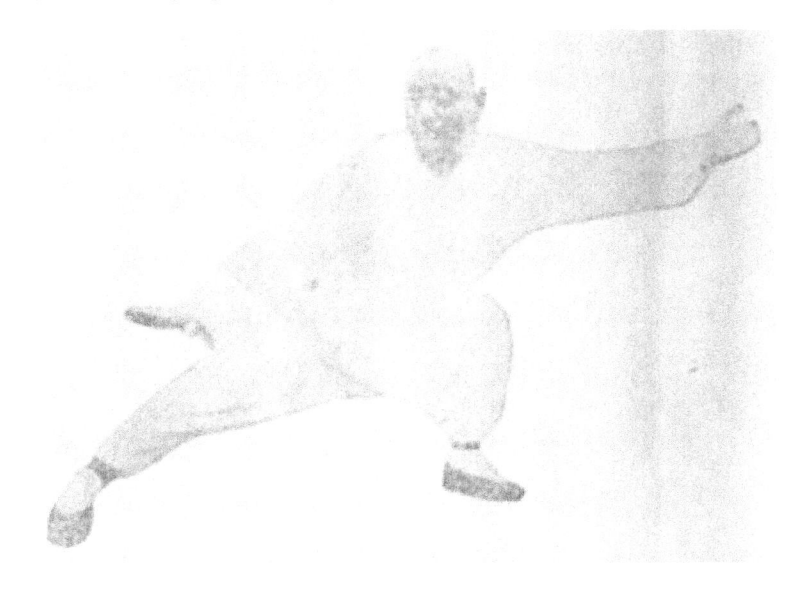

(25) Lift Hands Upward Posture (Picture 7)

(26) White Crane Spreads Wings (Picture 9)

(27) Grasp Sparrow's Tail, Single Whip (Picture 12)

(28) Needle at Sea Bottom (Picture 23)

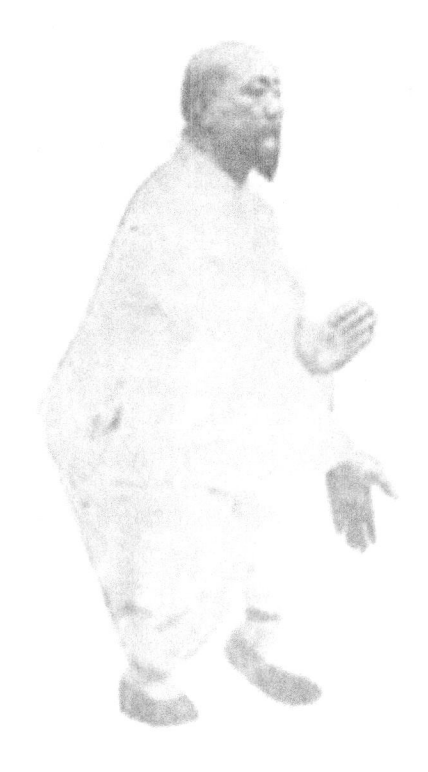

(29) Fan Through the Back (Picture 24)

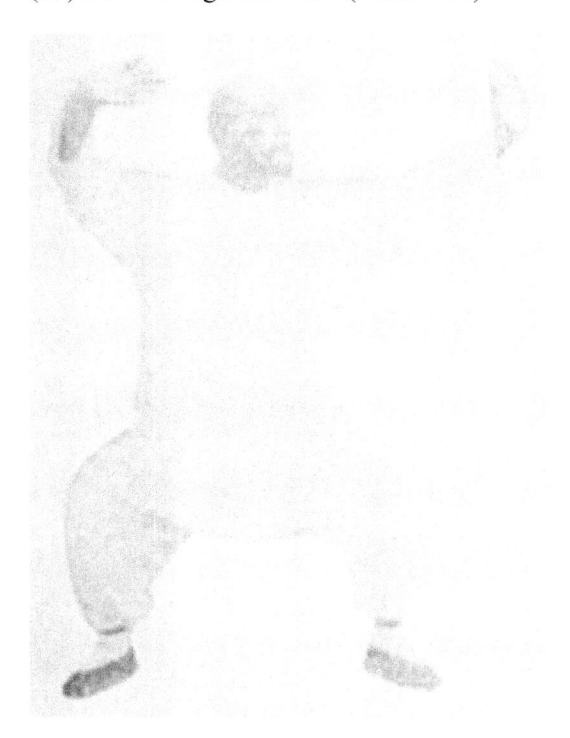

(30) Turn Body and Punch (Picture 25)

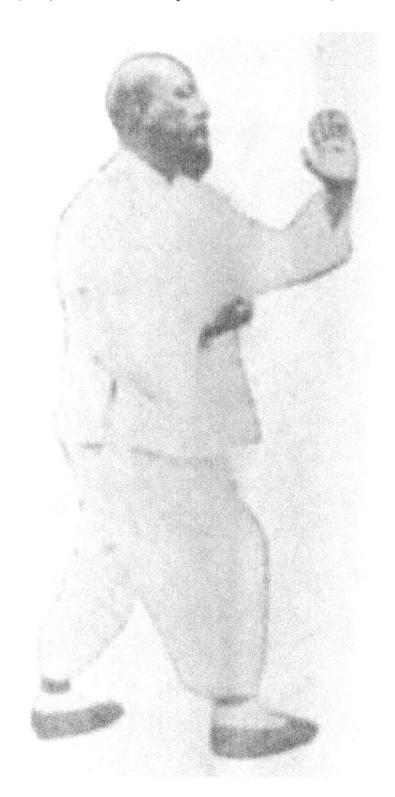

(31) Step Back, Deflect, Parry, and Punch (Picture 14)

(32) Ward Off, Grasp the Sparrow's Tail (Picture 4)

(33) Single Whip (Picture 6)

(34) Cloud Hands 1 (Picture 26)

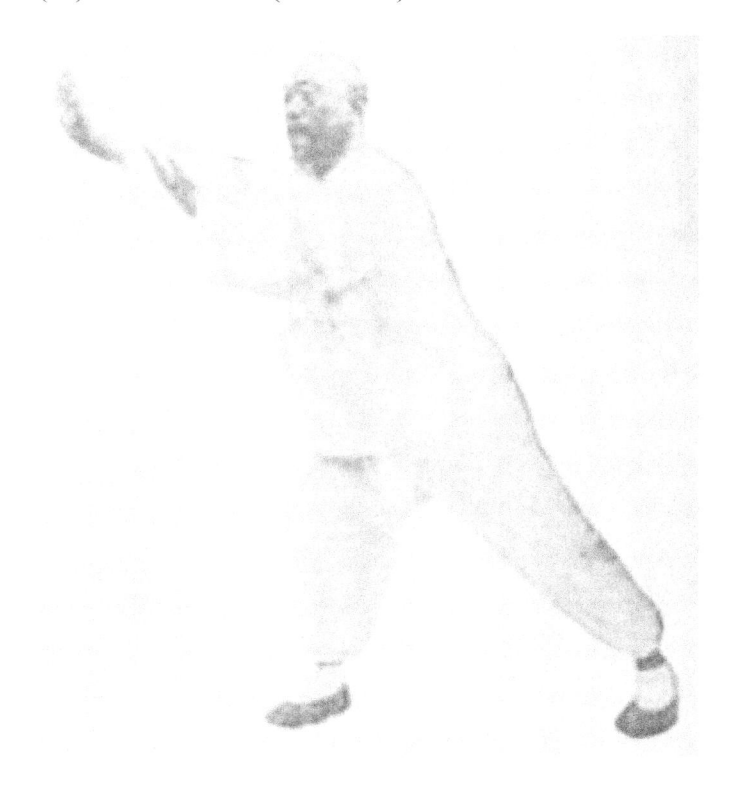

(35) Cloud Hands 2 (Picture 27)

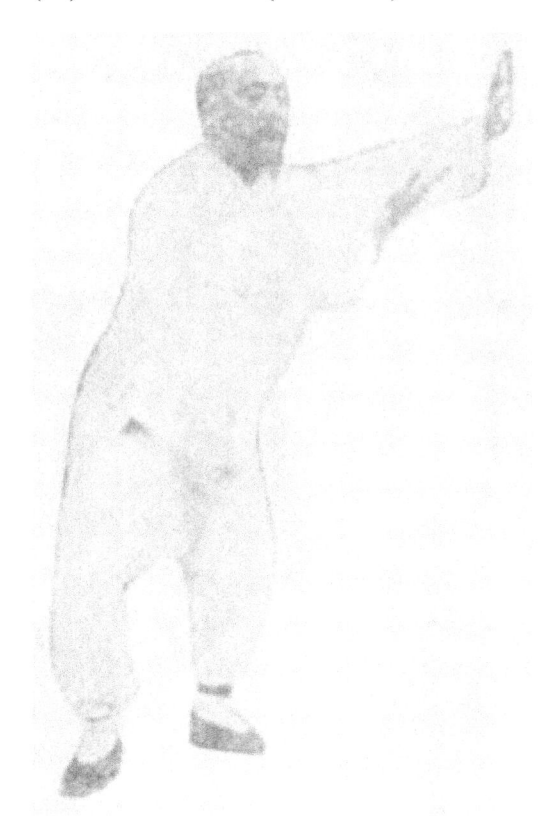

(36) High Pat on Horse (Left) (Picture 28)

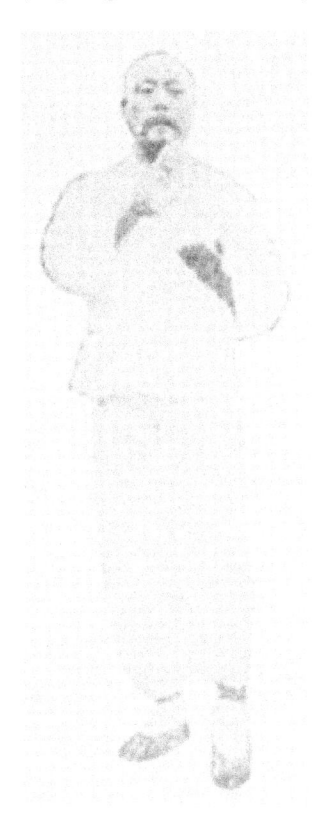

(37) Separate Leg (Right) (Picture 29)

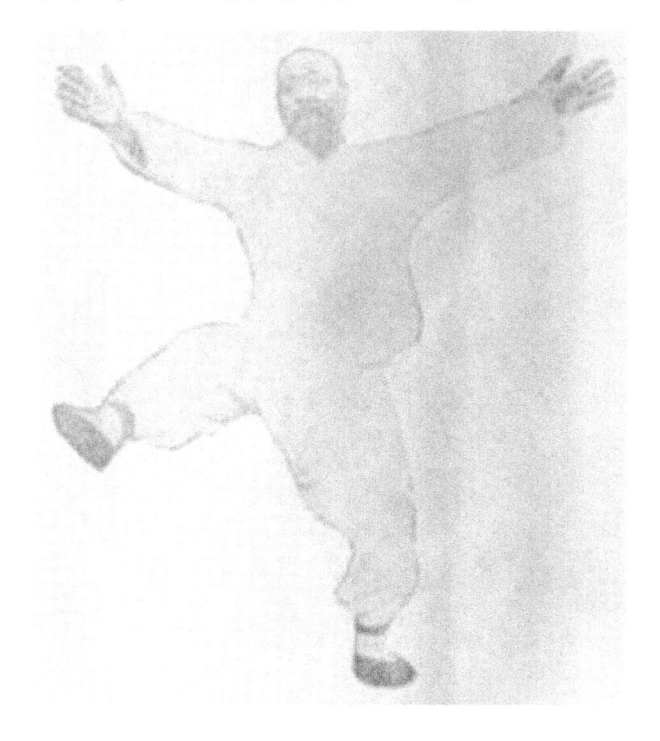

(38) High Pat on Horse (Right) (Picture 30)

(39) Separate Leg (Left) (Picture 31)

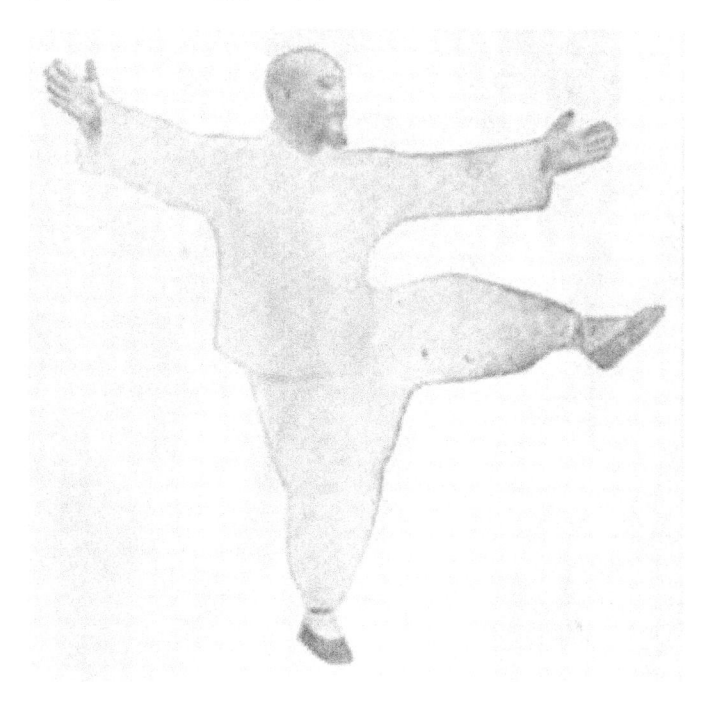

(40) Turn Body and Kick with Heel (1) (Picture 32) (*Note: The photo is missing.*)

(41) Turn Body and Kick with Heel (2) (Picture 33)

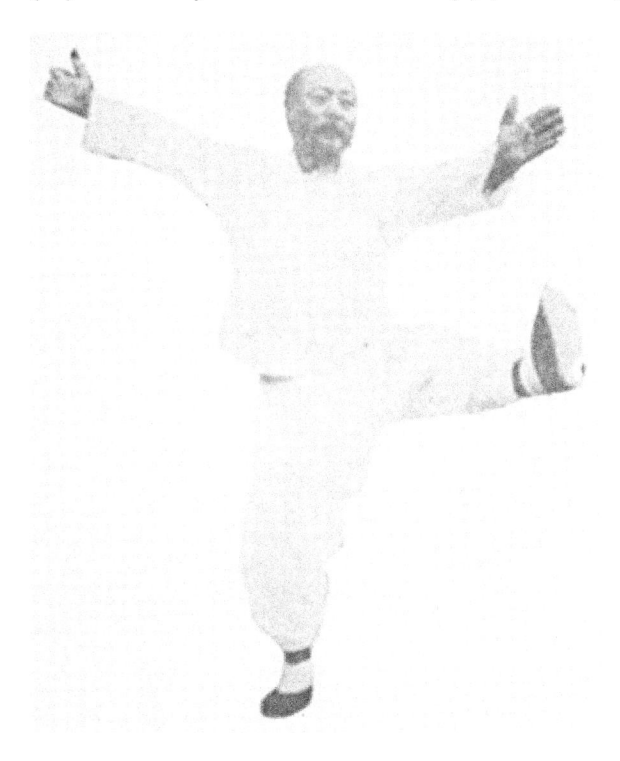

(42) Step Up and Punch Downward (Picture 34)

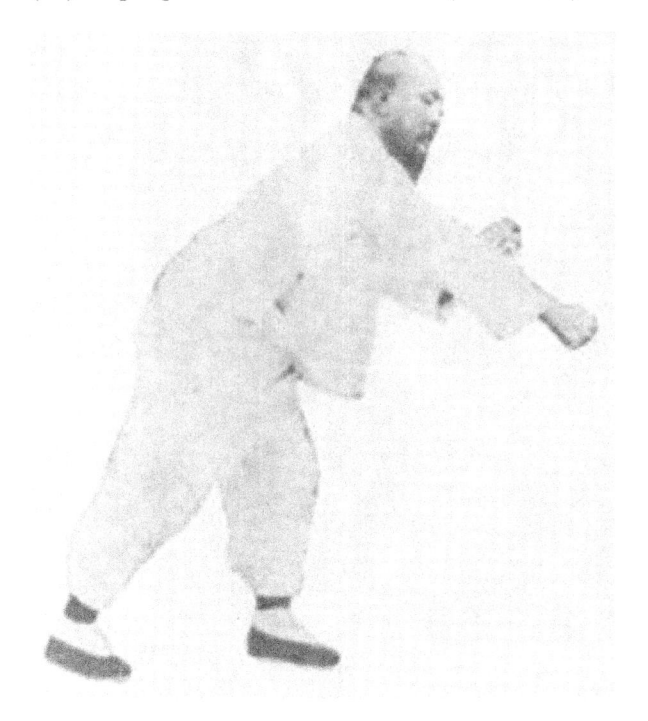

(43) Turn Body and Punch (Picture 25) (*Note: The photo is missing.*)

(44) Turn Body and Double Kick 1 (Picture 35)

(45) Turn Body and Double Kick 2 (Picture 36)

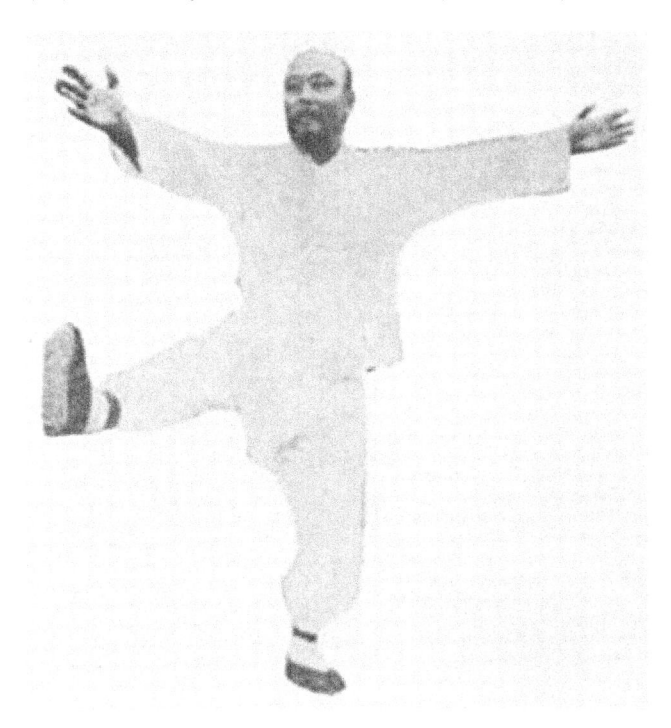

(46) Double Wind Sweeping Ears 1 (Picture 37) (*Note: The photo is missing.*)

(47) Double Wind Sweeping Ears 2 (Picture 38)

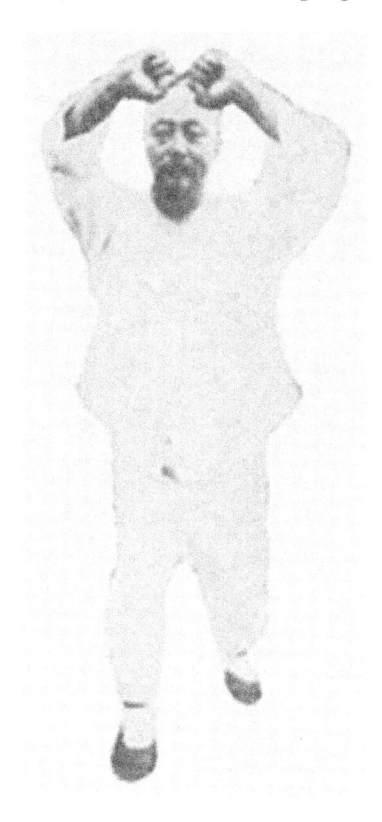

(48) Cover the Body and Kick (Picture 35)

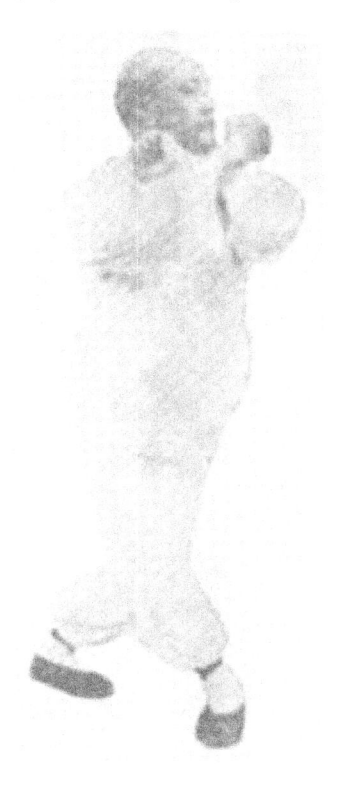

(49) Turn Around, Kick with Heel (Picture 33)

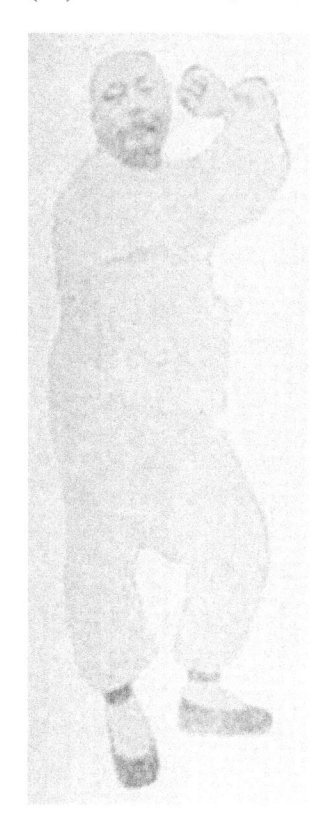

(50) Step Up and Deflect Downward, Punch (Picture 15)

(51) Closing and Sealing (Picture 16)

(52) Embrace Tiger and Return to Mountain (Picture 17)

(53) Brush Knee and Twist Step (Picture 11)

(54) Grasp the Bird's Tail (Picture 3)

(55) Diagonal Single Whip (Picture 20)

(56) Wild Horse Separates Mane (Left 1) (Picture 39)

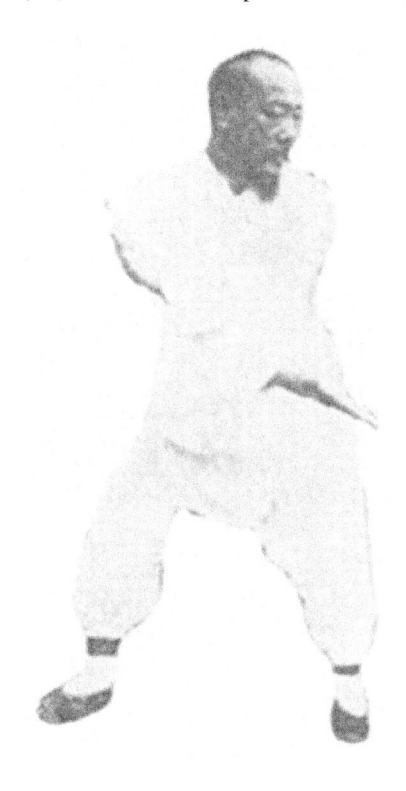

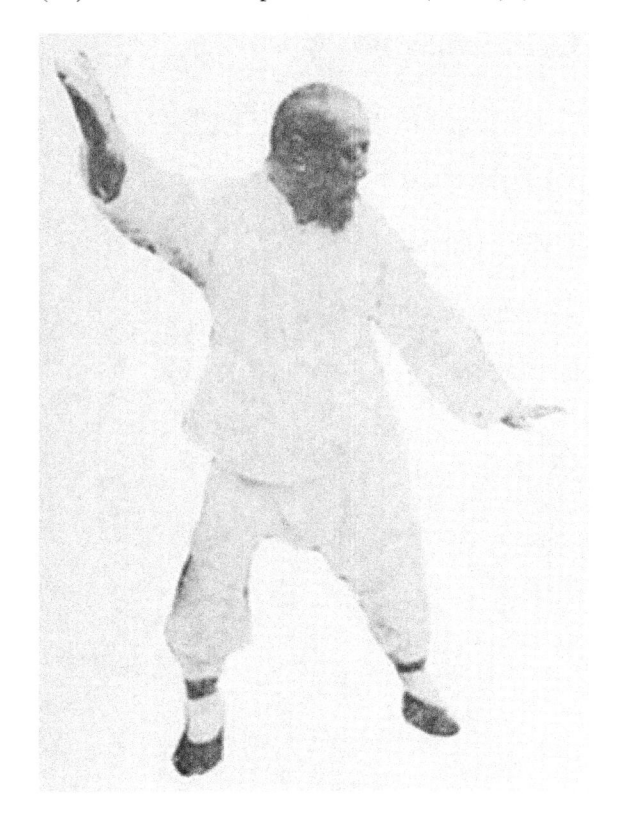

(57) Wild Horse Separates Mane (Left 2) (Picture 40)

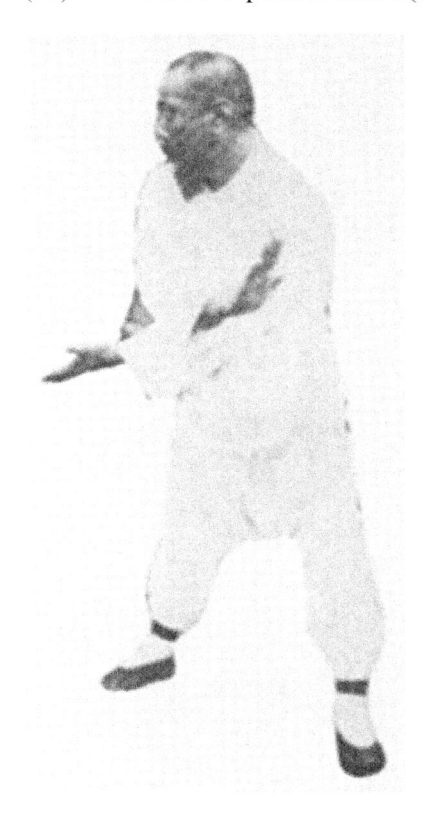

(58) Wild Horse Separates Mane (Right 1) (Picture 41)

(59) Wild Horse Separates Mane (Right 2) (Picture 42)

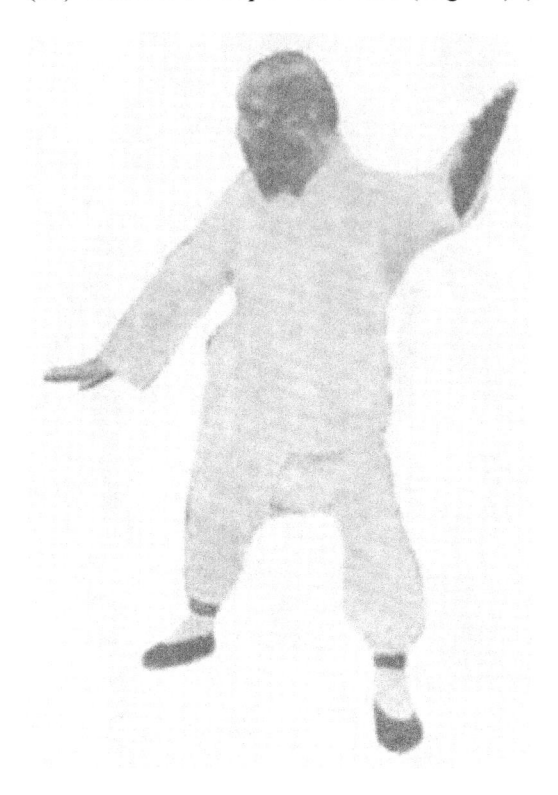

(60) Fair Lady Works Shuttles (Left) (Picture 43)

(61) Fair Lady Works Shuttles (Right) (Picture 44)

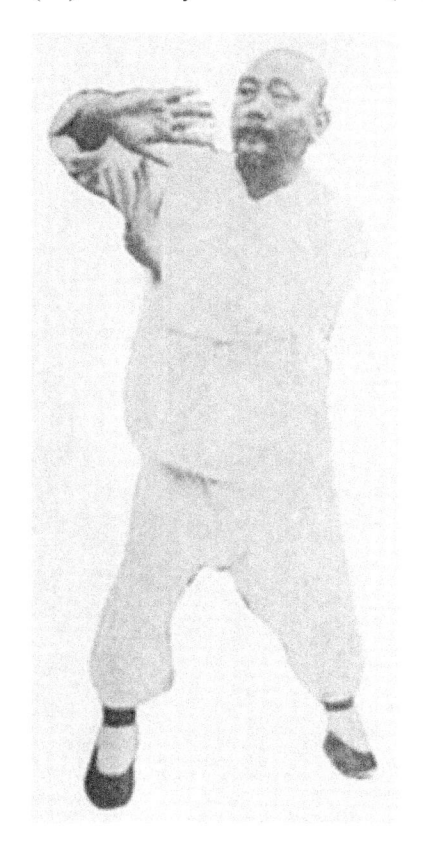

(62) Single Whip (Picture 6)

(63) Cloud Hands (Picture 26)

(64) Lower Stance (Picture 45)

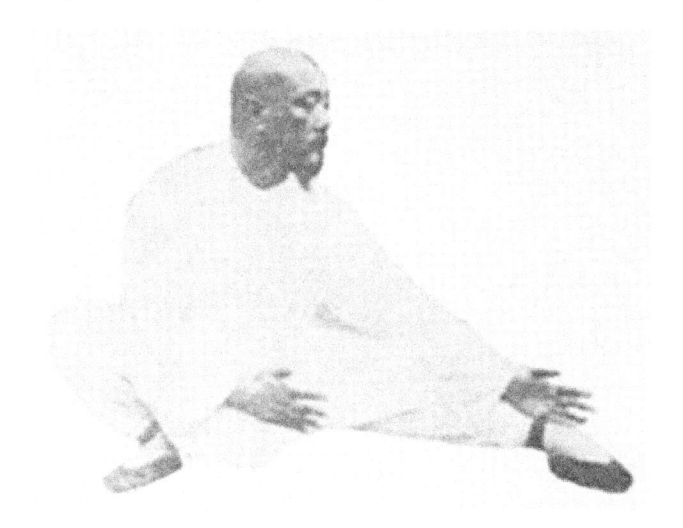

(65) Golden Rooster Stands on One Leg (Picture 46)

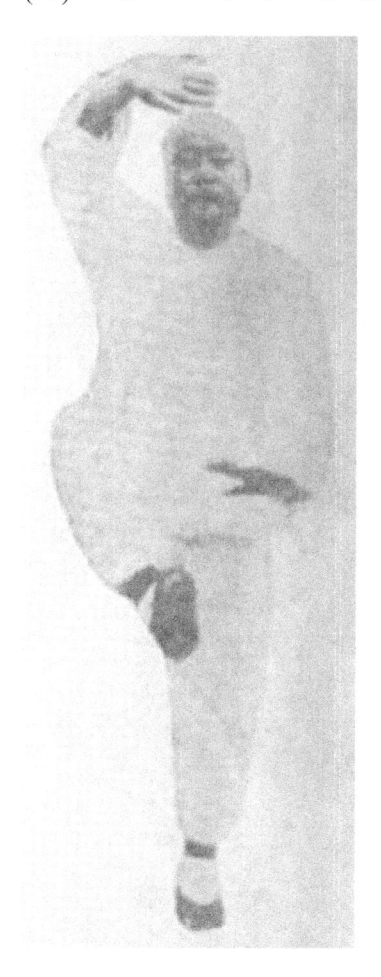

(66) Retreat and Repulse the Monkey (Picture 20)

(67) Slant Flying (Picture 22)

(68) Raise Hands and Step Up (Picture 7)

(69) White Crane Spreads Its Wings (Picture 10)

(70) Brush Knee Twist Step (Picture 11)

(71) Needle at Sea Bottom (Picture 23)

(72) Fan Through the Back (Picture 24)

(73) Step Forward, Deflect, Parry, and Punch (Picture 15)

(74) Step Forward and Grasp the Sparrow's Tail (Picture 4)

(75) Single Whip (Picture 6)

(76) Cloud Hands (Picture 26)

(77) High Pat on Horse (Picture 28)

(78) Palm Strike to the Face (Picture 47)

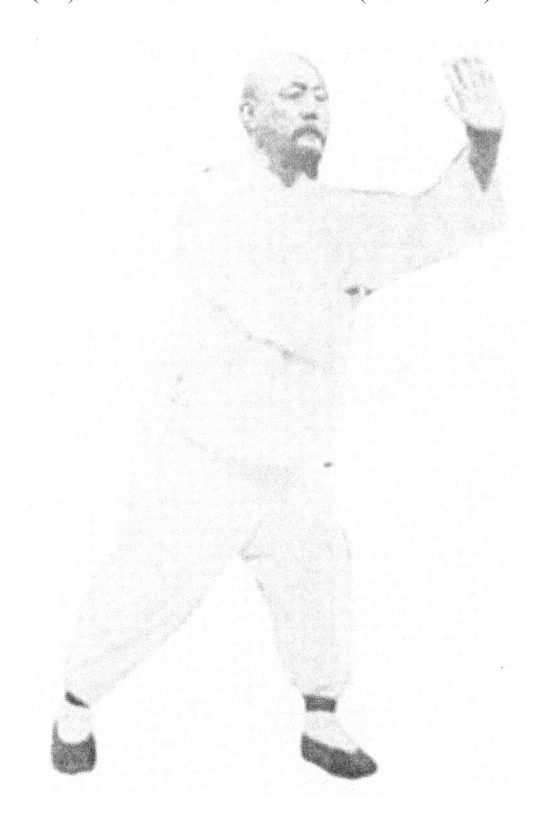

(79) Cross Hands and Swing the Lotus Kick (Picture 48)

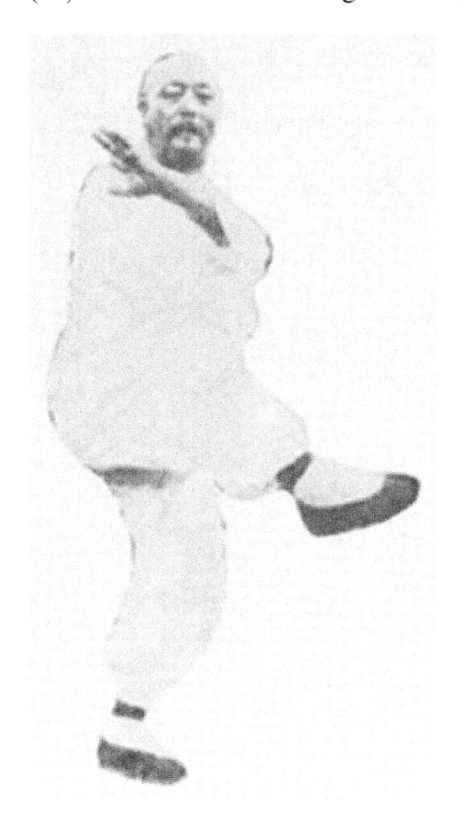

(80) Brush Knee and Strike the Groin (Picture 49)

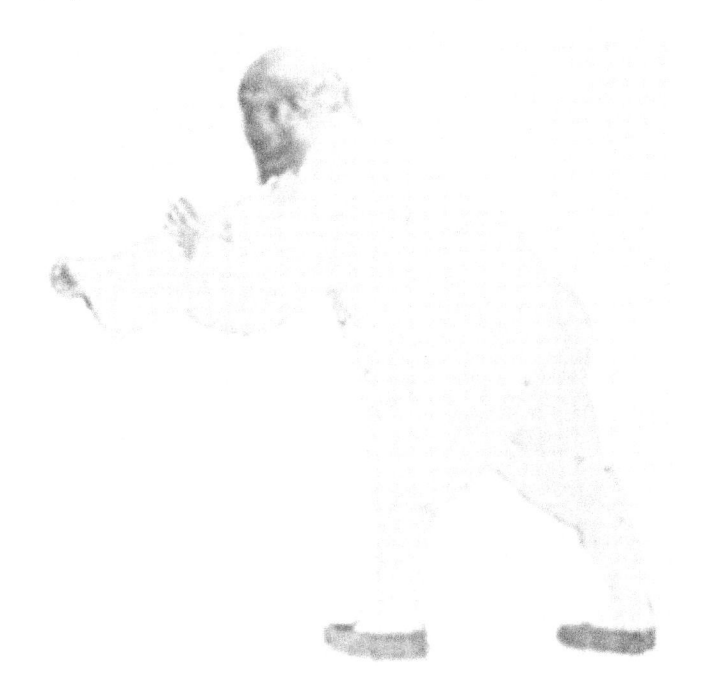

(81) Grasp the Sparrow's Tail in High Position (Picture 4)

(82) Single Whip (Picture 6)

(83) Lowering Movement (Picture 45)

(84) Step Up to Seven Stars (Picture 50)

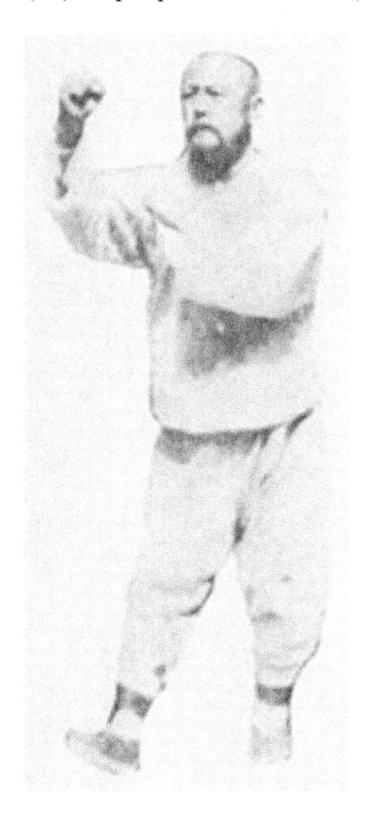

(85) Step Back and Ride the Tiger (Picture 51a and 51b)

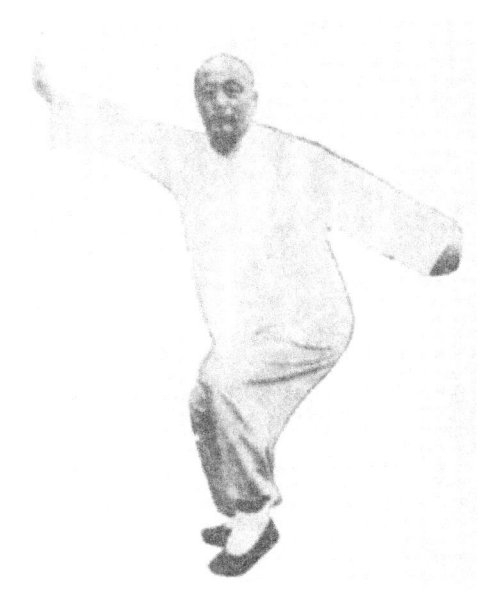

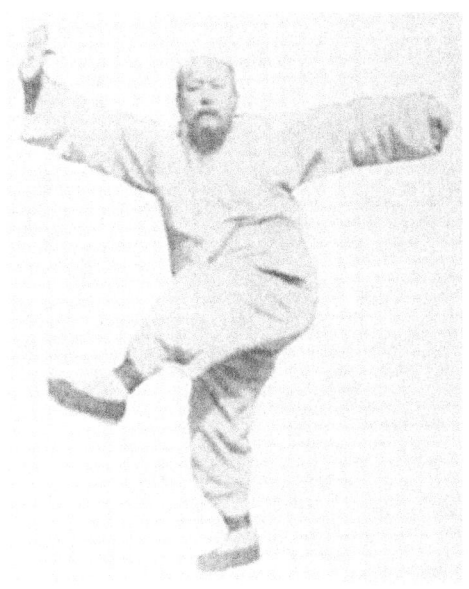

(86) Turn and Kick with Lotus Swing (Picture 52)

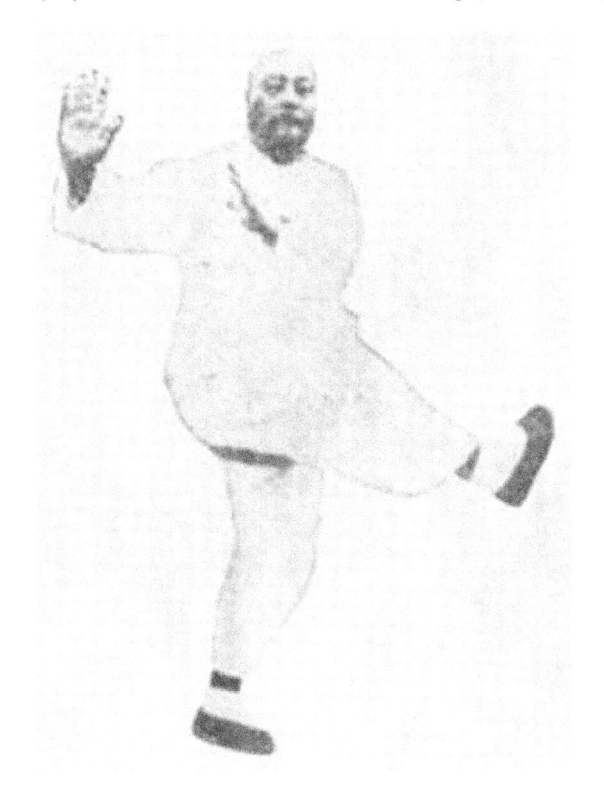

(87) Bend the Bow and Shoot the Tiger (Picture 53)

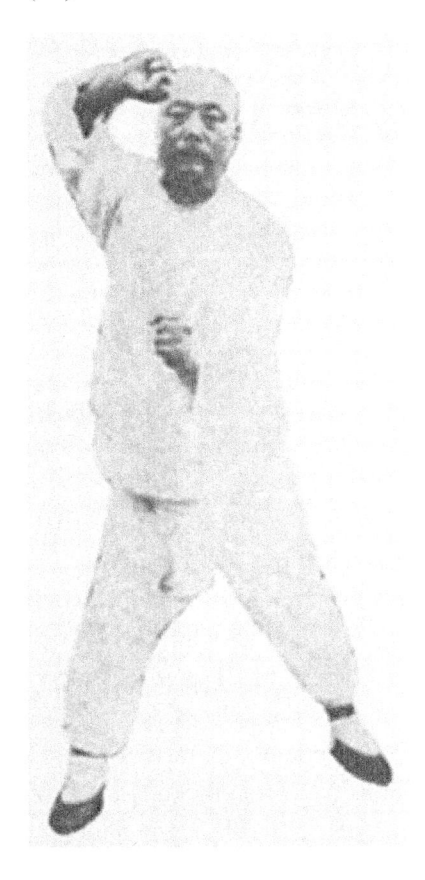

(88) Step Forward and Rise with High Pat on Horse (Picture 30)

(89) Palm Strike to the Face (Picture 47)

(90) Turn and Thrust Punch (Picture 25)

(91) Step Forward and Rise with High Pat on Horse (Picture 28)

(92) Step Forward and Grasp the Sparrow's Tail (Picture 4)

(93) Close Taijiquan (Picture 1)

Explanation of Taijiquan Push Hands and Equipment: Applying Science to the Study of Chinese Martial Arts

By Chu Minyi

Martial arts are practiced to engage the tendons and bones, to cultivate both the body and mind. Taijiquan, in particular, has the ability to cultivate and refine the body and mind, harmonize Qi and blood, cultivate temperament, and promote longevity by warding off illnesses. With prolonged practice, it becomes deeply engaging and enjoyable, making it an exceptional martial art. Its movements are gentle, and its postures are smooth. In terms of functionality, it can overcome strength with softness, conquer hardness with flexibility, achieve victory through lightness, and evade harm through adaptability. I have developed a strong passion for it, practicing it daily regardless of the weather. However, to further advance in martial arts, it is necessary to practice Pushing Hands, which requires at least two participants. The goal is to develop sensitivity throughout the entire body, maintaining a constant connection without detachment, and manifesting the sticky energy (nian jin) to achieve remarkable effects.

As I am unable to practice Pushing Hands with another person, I have devised alternative methods to supplement it. Through scientific principles, I have created two equipment: a stick and a ball, which serve as substitutes for Pushing Hands. This enables the scientificization of Chinese martial arts. These two objects can be utilized for the application of the eight techniques (Peng, Lu, Ji, An, Cai, Lie, Zhou, Kao) in Pushing Hands, simulating the interaction without detachment. Since their invention, they have attracted astonishment and admiration from sports and martial arts enthusiasts, both domestic and foreign. Now, I will explain their structures as follows.

Pole

First, create a pole that can rotate on its own. Attach one end of the stick with eight rubber bands, and the other ends are connected to an octagonal compartment or a cubic wooden frame. With this setup, the stick is suspended in the center of the compartment. If an external force disrupts its equilibrium, it will move in the direction of that force. When the force retreats, the equilibrium is restored. Thus, regardless of the force's direction from above, below, left, right, front, or back, various movements can be executed smoothly. Therefore, the eight techniques in Pushing Hands can be performed accordingly, just as in the two-person practice. The practitioner stands in front of or behind the stick, engaging in exercises that are equivalent to two-person Pushing Hands.

Taijiquan Pole Pictures

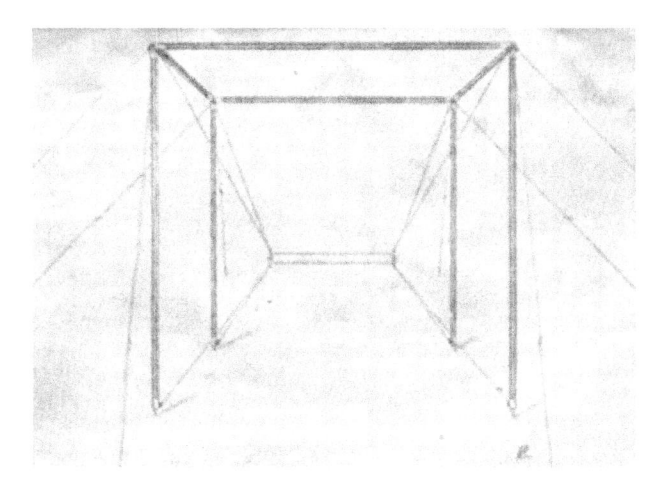

Taijiquan Pole Picture

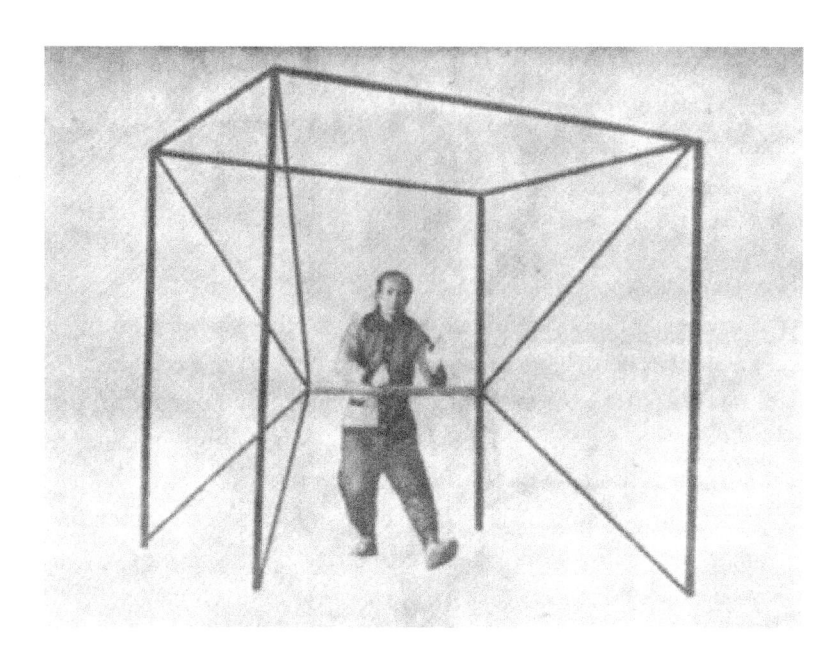

Taijiquan Pole Application One.

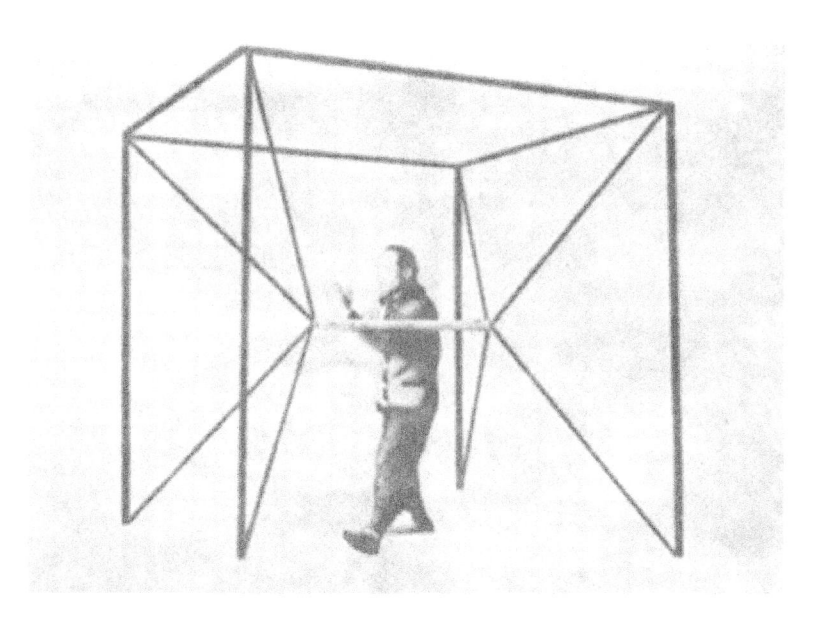

Taijiquan Pole Application Two.

82

Taijiquan Ball Pictures

The diameter of the ball is one and a half Chinese feet, weighing eighteen catties. It is made of copper and coated with nickel. It is suspended in the air by a rubber band. The height of the ball is at the level of a person's chest. Due to the attachment of the rubber band, it responds to external forces and moves in the direction of the applied force, be it up, down, left, right, or forward. It can rotate smoothly according to one's intention. When a person stands in front or behind the ball, they can perform various Taijiquan postures with ease. The eight techniques of push hands can also be demonstrated one by one. With these two objects, even when practicing alone, one can gradually progress in the profoundness of Taijiquan. It can be said that they are tools for the scientific development of Taijiquan.

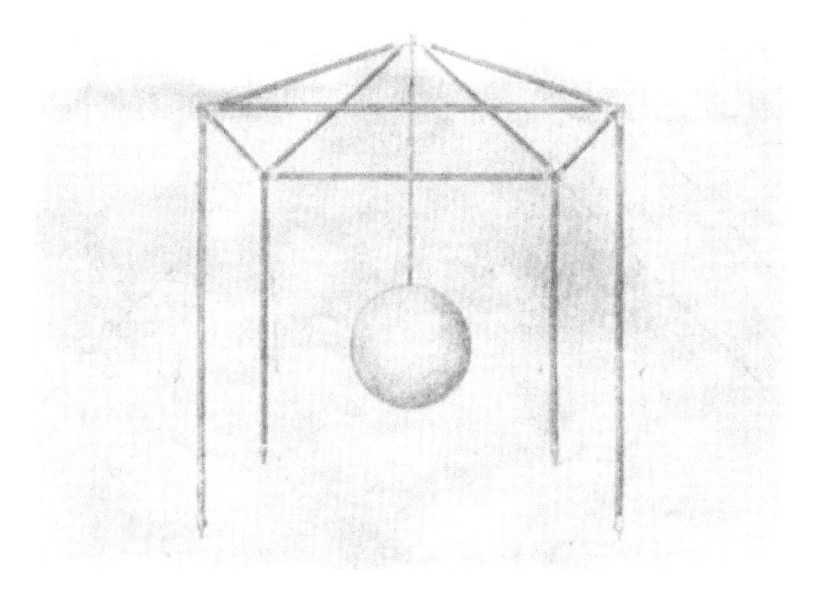

Picture of Taijiquan Ball

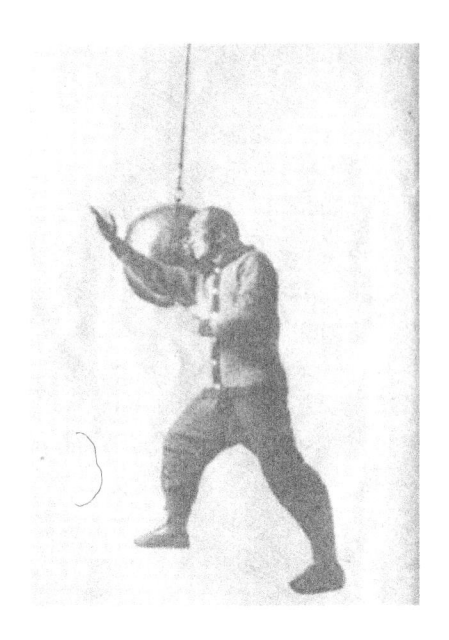

Taijiquan Ball Application One

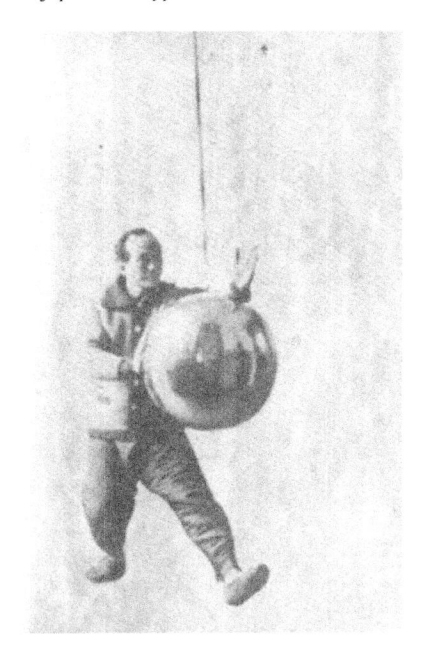

Taijiquan Ball Application Two

The above two types of equipment are constructed with the wisdom and knowledge of scientific application. This small invention, I dare not claim it to be a significant contribution to our nation's martial arts. However, our aim in promoting martial arts is indeed to make them scientific. By scientific, we mean that they should be adaptable to mechanics and psychology, emphasizing physiology and hygiene. Taijiquan's ability to overcome strength with gentleness, to conquer hardness with softness, is already known for its application of psychology and understanding of mechanics. Its stable postures, gentle movements, impartiality, and moderation are all manifestations of emphasizing physiology and hygiene. Therefore, it is not inappropriate to consider Taijiquan as a martial art that has undergone scientific development. However, should we not begin our promotion of martial arts with Taijiquan? This humble creation aims to make it accessible and beneficial to practitioners, serving as a starting point for the scientific development of our nation's martial arts.

Regarding the belief in Taijiquan, my dedication to daily practice has become even more diligent. However, after the completion of the solo form, I desired to continue with pushing hands. Often, I encountered difficulties in practicing with just one partner. As a result, the invention of pushing hands equipment emerged to serve as a substitute for an opponent.

The motivation behind inventing pushing hands equipment originated during my time in Beiping. Mr. Tan Zhongkui provided me with a clue. When Mr. Wu introduced him to me, he was already highly proficient in Taijiquan. Unfortunately, he later discontinued his practice, which has been a great loss. He gave me some hints, occasionally mentioning the possibility of using equipment to practice this art. At that time, as a novice, I couldn't fully comprehend his suggestion. Last year, during my trip to Europe for health research, I continued practicing on the boat every day and even taught Mr. Chen Zongcheng, a fellow passenger (he is currently a secretary at the International Labor Bureau, I wonder if he still practices).

During that time, I would perform boxing and sword forms alone on the boat but never had the opportunity for pushing hands. Sometimes, I would stand by the edge of the boat, rubbing my hands against the railings, simulating pushing hands movements. I imagined how wonderful it would be if the railing could rotate freely, allowing for movement in all directions. This ideal led to the invention of the pushing hands stick. Its structure involves creating a wooden pole that can spin on its own axis, with four rubber bands attached to each end to maintain balance. The four rubber bands on each end are analogous to the four muscles of our eyes, enabling free movement in various directions. The attachment of rubber bands to the pushing hands pole serves a similar purpose.

As for the Taiji ball, it evolved from the sandbags used in ancient China. However, while the sandbags were struck with fists, the Taiji ball utilizes the power of the arms, shoulders, chest, and back to push it. The sandbag was suspended with ropes, while the Taiji ball is suspended in mid-air with elastic bands, allowing for dynamic movement in all directions. It is agile and responsive.

The third type of pushing hands equipment has a relatively simpler structure. Although these three types of pushing hands equipment benefit the practice of pushing hands and have been extensively practiced, they can also help to discover the Eight Gates (Peng, Lu, Ji, An, Cai, Lie, Zhou, Kao) and the Five Elements (Jin, Tui, Gu, Pan, Ting) within Taijiquan. However, no matter what, I still believe that it is not as sensitive as pushing hands between individuals.

Pushing hands equipment is always controlled by humans and passive in nature. It moves in the direction dictated by human force. Its response is limited to returning in the opposite direction. On the other hand, pushing hands between individuals involves both parties having intentions. While I may want to take a passive role, sometimes the other person may also want to be passive. This is why the concept of "listening energy" in pushing hands is easier to grasp with equipment but more challenging when it comes to interactions between individuals. However, during the learning process, equipment is also an indispensable and excellent assistant. As everything progresses from easy to difficult, it is advisable to first become proficient in using equipment that facilitates understanding of "listening energy" before advancing to the more challenging practice of "listening energy" between individuals. This is the reason for inventing these three types of equipment. Fellow practitioners in the martial arts community have praised their effectiveness, expressing admiration and envy. I also highly value them myself and hope to promote these equipment, replacing all intense and forceful exercises. Although intense and forceful exercises have their own merits, their drawbacks outweigh the benefits, resulting in a net loss. These three types of equipment, on the other hand, are gentle, soft, and beneficial to health. Even individuals who are weak or fragile can engage in their practice. This is their greatest advantage compared to other forms of exercise that are primarily intended for the young and strong. Recently, I have been dedicating a significant amount of time, ranging from ten minutes to half an hour or even an hour, to daily practice using these three Taijiquan pushing hands equipment. I have experienced rapid progress, so I am eager to introduce them to those who haven't yet learned Taijiquan, so they too can practice and exercise, strengthening their muscles and reducing physical discomfort. This will contribute to enhancing their health and happiness.

Applications of Taijiquan Pole

1. Hand Training

Stand in front of the pole, facing east and back to the west. Sit on the right leg with the left foot pointing forward and the heel touching the ground. Place the left hand flat on the pole, with the back of the hand facing upwards. (See picture one)

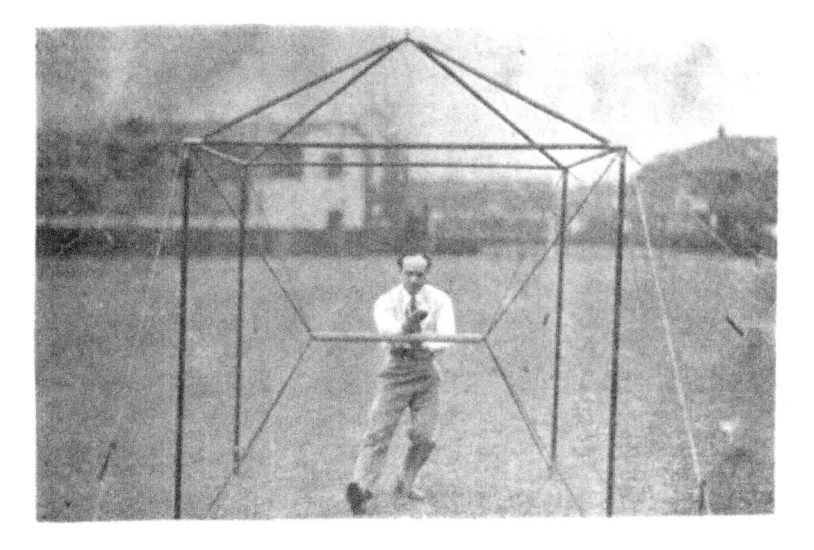

Using the left hand, push the pole. First, move towards the east, then turn to the south, west, and finally north, forming a circular shape. This circular motion is limited to a plane. After several repetitions, reverse the movement. Sit on the left leg with the right foot pointing forward and the heel touching the ground. Place the right hand flat on the pole, with the back of the hand facing upwards and the palm touching the pole. Using the right hand, push the pole. First, turn to the east, then to the north, west, and finally south; forming a circular shape on the same plane. The palm should face upwards, and the back of the hand should touch the pole. This is the first form of placing the hand on the pole.

The second form is similar in hand and foot placement as well as sitting posture to the first form. However, during the push, if using the left hand, the left hand turns upward first to the south and then downward to the north. If using the right hand, the right hand turns upward first to the north and then downward to the south, forming a horizontal circular shape.

The third form maintains the same hand, foot, and sitting posture as before. However, during the push, the hand turns upward first to the east and then downward to the west, or it can be reversed by turning upward to the west and then downward to the east, forming a vertical circular shape.

These three forms create three types of circular shapes: (1) a circular shape on the same plane, (2) a circular shape on a horizontal plane, and (3) a circular shape on a vertical plane. At the same time, there are six directions: up, down, east (front), south (left), west (back), and north (right). The three circular shapes combined form a sphere.

However, all the above descriptions are based on using the left hand while sitting on the right leg, or using the right hand while sitting on the left leg. With sufficient practice, one can freely switch between them. For example, when using the left hand, one can also sit on the left leg, and when using the right hand, one can sit on the right leg. After becoming familiar with single-handed movements, progress to using both hands to push, creating three circular shapes and changing in six directions. The sitting posture can also be freely adjusted between the legs.

Once proficiency is achieved in hand movements on the pole, one can further interchange the positions of the hand and the pole. Place the hand under the pole, with the back of the hand facing downwards and the palm touching the pole. Then, have the back of the hand touch the pole, with the palm facing downwards. The sitting posture can be on the left or right leg, also interchangeable. When pushing, also create three circular shapes and six directions. In this way, the hand can alternately be on the pole or below the pole, lifting and flipping freely. The movements transition from simplicity to complexity and from slowness to agility. Upon closer observation, the hand and the pole appear to stick together, and neither separated nor forcefully pressed, but fused in one place.

2. Wrist Training (Commonly Known as Forearm)

Stand in front of the pole, facing east and with the back towards the west. Sit on the right leg. The left foot is placed forward, with the heel touching the ground. Place the left wrist flat on the pole, palm facing downwards. Using the left wrist, push the pole. First, move towards the east, then turn to the south, west, and finally north, forming a circular shape on the same plane. At the same time, switch to the right wrist, following the same method as hand training. Perform three variations to create three circular shapes and six directions. The same principles can be applied for other wrists.

When the wrist is on the pole, the palm faces downwards. When the wrist is below the pole, the palm faces upwards. The direction of the wrist changes with the rotation of the palm, allowing for smooth and circular movements, similar to a spinning axle. When placing the wrist on the pole, the palm can alternately face upwards or downwards, and the same applies when the wrist is below the pole. For example, when the left wrist is flat on the pole with the palm facing downwards, push towards the east and turn to the south. As the hand and wrist are tilted to the side of the pole, the palm faces south. When moving from south to west, the palm faces upwards. Upon reaching the north, the palm faces downwards, and the wrist also moves downwards. Conversely, when the palm of the left wrist facing downwards, push towards the east and turn to the north. The palm also faces north. When moving from north to west, the hand and wrist are tilted to the side of the pole, and the palm faces south. Upon reaching the south, the palm faces upwards, and the wrist moves upwards. When moving from south to east, the wrist rotates inward, and the palm faces downwards to return to the original position. This specifically refers to the left wrist. If practicing with the right wrist, simply change the pushing direction. The same principles can be easily applied to other wrists.

3. Arm Training (Commonly Known as Upper Arm, from Shoulder to Wrist)

The training method for the arms is similar to what was mentioned above and does not require further elaboration. However, practicing the arms is not as easy as the wrists.

The three methods described above should be clearly distinguished during practice to avoid confusion. In other words, when practicing the hands, the focus is solely on the relationship between the hands and the pole. When practicing the wrists or arms, the focus is solely on the relationship between the wrists or arms and the pole. However, at the same time, the movements should be coordinated. During the pushing motion, the hand, wrist, and arm should all rub against the pole, activating and circulating the muscles, bones, and blood in the upper body. This rubbing technique between the skin and the pole is similar to Chinese massage therapy and Western massage techniques. Through the movement of the muscles and bones, the internal body can also experience the massage effect. Massage therapy requires another person to perform the rubbing, while electric massagers use electricity for the rubbing. Both are passive methods. However, using equipment for rubbing, as in this case, is an automatic method. We often see elderly individuals who frequently experience discomfort and soreness in their muscles and bones, requiring others to pat their backs or massage their chests. This is because they did not pay attention to exercise and movement during their prime years, resulting in the need for passive massage techniques involving human or electric force. Pushing the hands against the pole not only exercises the arms but also helps mobilize and stretch the back, waist, chest, and ribs. Now, let's further discuss it in the following sections.

4. Back Training

Stand with the pole against the back, making contact with it. Sit on the left leg or right leg. The left foot or right foot is positioned forward with the heel touching the ground. The body slightly leans forward, assuming a bowing posture. The pole rides along the back, and the chest is pushed forward. The pole then descends. (See Picture 2)

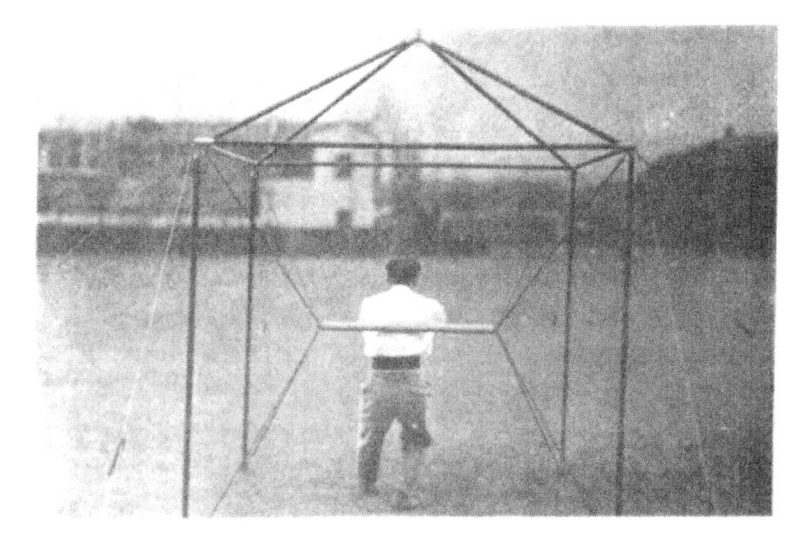

This exercise embodies the intention of Taijiquan to contain the chest and lift the back. By straightening the chest and bowing the back, the pole smoothly moves up and down without detachment. Initially, the pole rides up and down in a straight line. With practice, the pole can ascend from the left side of the back while descending from the right side, or ascend from the right side and descend from the left side, forming a circular motion. The waist also rotates as a result of the body's lateral movement. Furthermore, there is another method of back training where the body bends forward, curving the back under the pole. The back and the pole form parallel lines, allowing the back to connect with the pole. Both arms are extended and swung left and right, causing the pole to rotate like a wheel on the left and right sides of the back.

5. Waist and Rib Training

Stand sideways next to the pole. Place the pole below the left rib. Sit on the left leg, with the right foot forward and the heel on the ground. Lean the body to the right. The pole rises along the left rib. Then turn to the left. The pole descends. When placing the pole below the right rib, sit on the right leg, with the left foot forward and the heel on the ground. Lean the body to the left. The pole rises along the right rib. Then turn to the right. The pole descends. When training the left rib, you can also sit on the right leg. When training the right rib, you can sit on the left leg. In this way, the pole rubs against the waist and ribs wherever it goes.

6. Chest Training

Stand facing the pole with your chest tightly pressed against it. Begin by sitting on your left leg, bending your chest forward. As you do this, the pole moves downward. Lean your chest backward, and the pole moves upward. You can also perform this exercise while sitting on your right leg, rotating your chest from left to right. This allows the pole to move in a circular motion, either from upper left to lower right or upper right to lower left. The rotation of the waist follows the movement of the chest from side to side. Another variation of this exercise involves sitting on both legs, assuming the posture of Single Whip in Taijiquan, which also emphasizes the importance of maintaining a lifted chest and an upright back.

Applications of Taijiquan Ball

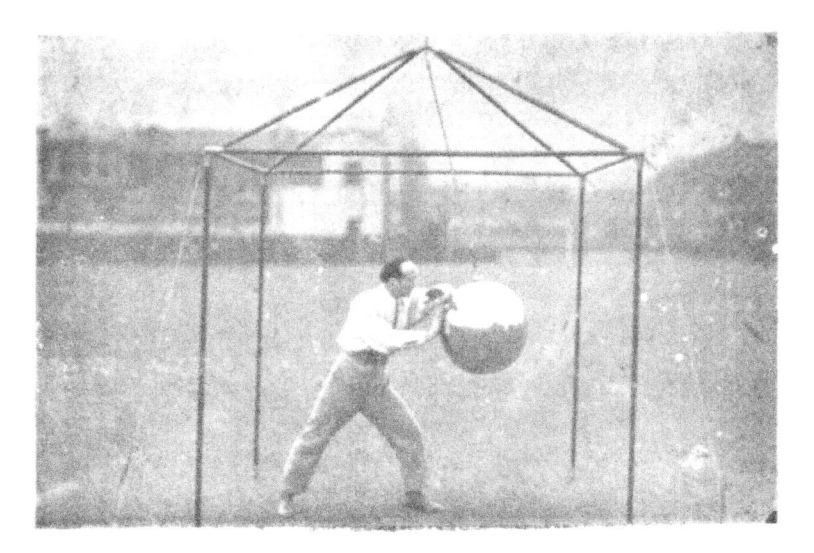

(Part A) Single Arm Training

1. Stand facing the ball, oriented to the east. Sit on your left leg with your left foot forward, heel touching the ground. Your right upper arm and hand should be in contact with the side of the ball, assuming a palm-touching-ball position. Slowly raise your hand upward and place it on top of the ball, then continue moving northward and downward, forming a horizontal circular motion. When your hand is moving upward, the palm should be touching the ball. As it moves from top to north, the back of the hand should be in contact with the ball. When it reaches the bottom of the ball, the hand turns outward, and the palm again touches the bottom of the ball. After repeating this several times, you can change direction. The upper arm moves from north to up, with the back of the hand touching the ball. When the hand reaches the top of the ball, the upper arm moves

to the side of the ball. As it moves from south to down, the hand rotates inward, and the palm touches the ball. Repeat this process several times. Then you can sit on your right leg and use your left hand, following the same exercise method as with the right hand, forming a horizontal circular motion. After becoming proficient in practice, you can also train the left hand by sitting on your left leg, or train the right hand by sitting on your right leg.

2. Stand facing the ball, oriented to the east. Sit on your left leg with your right foot forward, heel touching the ground. Your right hand and upper arm should also be in contact with the side of the ball, assuming a palm-touching-ball position. Slowly raise your hand from east to up, then rotate to the west and downward. The upper arm should always be in contact with the half sphere, forming a vertical circular motion. After several repetitions, you can change direction, starting from below and moving westward, then rotating upward and eastward. When training the left hand, sit on your right leg and perform two circular motions, similar to the right hand. It is also possible to train the left hand while sitting on your left leg and the right hand while sitting on your right leg. This depends on the understanding and comprehension of the practitioner.

3. Stand facing the ball, oriented to the east. Sit back with the weight on your left leg with your right foot forward, heel touching the ground. Your right hand and upper arm should be in contact with the bottom of the ball. Gradually move your hand from east to north, then rotate west to south, forming a flat circular motion. After several repetitions, you can also change direction, moving from east to south, and then rotating west to

north, creating another flat circular motion. When training the left hand, sit on your right leg with your left foot forward, following the directions mentioned above. Perform two types of flat circular motions. It is also possible to train the left hand while sitting on your left leg and the right hand while sitting on your right leg.

(Part B) Training Both Arms

1. Stand facing the ball, oriented to the east. Sit on your left leg or right leg. The left or right foot should be forward with the heel touching the ground. Hold both hands in a hugging position, embracing the ball. Start with the right upper arm and hand, creating a vertical circular motion from top to west, then rotating down to the east. As the right hand moves from top to west, the left upper arm and hand should move from bottom to west, rotating up to the east. Repeat this circular motion.

2. Stand in a posture similar to the first stance, with the hands and feet positioned in the same way. However, this time, both upper arms and hands perform two identical vertical circular motions, but in different orientations. For example, the left upper arm and hand move from top to east, then rotate down to the west, while at the same time, the right upper arm and hand move from top to west, then rotate down to the east. This may be difficult at first, as our nerves find it challenging to coordinate different movements for each hand. For instance, when the right hand clenches into a fist, and the left hand remains flat on a table, it is difficult to make the right hand strike the table while the left hand rubs it simultaneously. Often, there is hesitation, resulting in both hands either striking the table or rubbing it. This is due to the limited capacity of our nerves to focus on

multiple actions at once. However, with prolonged practice, both hands can perform different movements simultaneously, and their actions can be in harmony. Moving the hands in the left-right direction around the ball is easier, while moving them in the up-down direction is more challenging due to the obstruction of the hanging string at the top of the ball. Therefore, in mixed practice exercises, one hand can move in the left-right direction, forming a vertical or horizontal circular motion, while the other hand remains in contact with the bottom of the ball, creating a flat circular motion. When training both arms, you can freely switch between sitting on your left leg and right leg. The body can lean forward to adopt an attacking posture or lean backward to assume a sitting posture. When adopting an attacking posture, the body leans forward with the left knee bent, aligning the tips of the left toes, left knee, and nose in a straight line, while the right leg extends backward like a supporting pillar. This is called "left substantial, right insubstantial." When assuming a sitting posture, sit on your right leg, with the left leg forward and the left heel touching the ground. This is called "right substantial, left insubstantial." In this way, the body moves back and forth, and the waist also moves.

In the first exercise of training with a single arm, when training the right arm, the palm and upper arm tightly adhere to the south side of the ball (i.e., the side). Now, place it on the opposite side of the ball, which is the north side. The back of the hand should be in contact with the ball. In this way, the ball is positioned to the right of the body, not facing directly in front. When training the left arm, the same applies. When performing the pushing movement, both arms create two vertical circular motions: (1) from top to east, rotating down to the west, and (2) from top to west, rotating down to the east. You can also freely switch between sitting on the leg.

Since it is not possible to practice on the top of the ball where the hanging string is, the left and right corners on top of the ball can be utilized. The training method is as follows: Sit on your right leg, place the left upper arm on the left corner of the ball, and rotate the hand and upper arm forward and then retract them backward. Create a diagonal or partially vertical and horizontal circular motion from top to west, rotating down to the east. This circular motion can also be performed from top to east, rotating down to the west. There are two directions. When practicing, pay attention to making the arms rotate like the axles of a wheel. Similarly, the right upper arm can also perform the same exercise on the right corner. You can sit on your left leg or right leg for this practice.

(Part C) Shoulder Training

1. Stand facing the ball, oriented to the east. Sit on your left leg or right leg, with the left or right foot forward and the heel touching the ground. Both hands assume a hugging posture, embracing the ball. Begin by making a vertical circular motion with the right arm and hand, moving from up to west and then down to east. While the right hand moves from up to west, the left arm and hand simultaneously move from down to west and then up to east. These circular motions are performed interchangeably.

2. Stand in the same position and leg stance as in the first exercise. However, this time, both arms and hands perform two vertical circular motions, but with different orientations. For instance, the left arm and hand move from up to east and then down to west, while the right arm and hand move from up to west and then down to

east. Initially, this may be challenging, but with practice, it becomes more proficient. Our nervous system finds it exceptionally difficult to coordinate different directional movements with both hands. For example, if you clench your right hand into a fist and keep your left hand flat on a table, it's challenging to make the right hand strike the table while the left hand rubs against it simultaneously. Often, there is hesitation, and both hands end up striking the table or rubbing against it. This is because our nerves can only focus on one area at a time. However, with prolonged practice, both hands can perform different movements simultaneously with ease. It is easier to move both hands from left to right or right to left around the ball, but more difficult to move them from top to bottom or bottom to top due to the obstruction of the ball's top attachment rope. Therefore, in mixed exercise forms, one hand can move from left to right or right to left to form a vertical or horizontal circular motion, while the other hand remains flat against the bottom of the ball, forming a planar circular motion. When training both arms, you can freely switch between sitting on the left leg and the right leg. By leaning forward, you adopt an attacking posture, while leaning backward, you assume a sitting posture. In the attacking posture, bend your left knee forward, aligning the tips of your left foot, left knee, and nose on a straight line, and extend your right leg backward, resembling a supporting pillar. This represents the left being substantial and the right being insubstantial. In the sitting posture, sit on the right leg, extend the left leg forward, and place the left heel on the ground. This represents the right being substantial and the left being insubstantial. In this way, the waist also moves due to the sudden forward and backward shifts of the body.

To practice the first form of single-arm exercise, when training the right arm, place the palm and arm tightly against the south side of the ball (the side). Now, position it opposite the south side of the ball (the north side), with the back of the hand against the ball. This way, the ball is located to the right side of the body, no longer facing directly. The same applies when training the left arm. When pushing, perform two vertical circular motions: (1) From up to east, then down to west, and (2) From up to west, then down to east. You can freely switch between sitting on the leg.

Since practicing at the top of the ball, where it is attached to the rope, is not possible, the left and right corners on the top of the ball can be utilized. To practice, start by sitting on the right leg, place the left arm on the left corner of the ball, and rotate the hand and arm forward and then retract it. Perform a diagonal or vertical and horizontal mixed circular motion from up to east, then down to west. This circular motion can also be performed from up to west, then down to east. During the exercise, pay attention to making the arms resemble the turning axis of a wheel. The right arm can also practice the same exercise on the right corner of the ball. You can sit on the left leg or right leg interchangeably.

Taijiquan Hand Training on the Ball

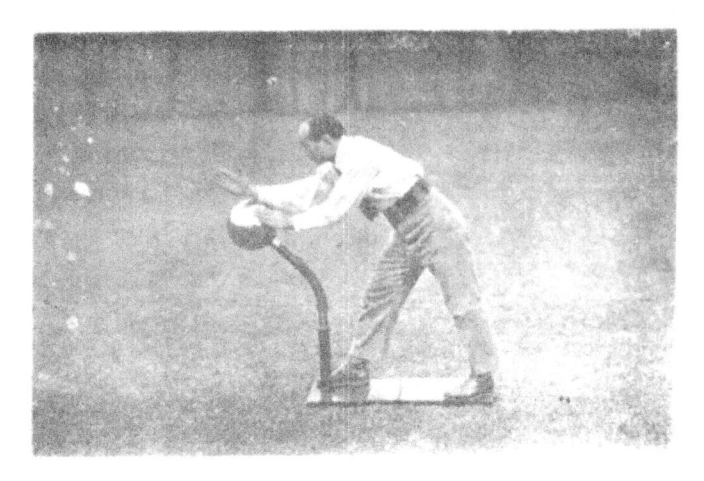

For those who specialize in exercising the arms, the structure consists of a ball with a diameter of about eight to nine inches. A pole with a spring is set up, and the ball is placed on top of the pole. The pole is erected on flat ground or a board, with a person standing at one end. They lean forward and use their hand or arm to push the ball. The ball can also rotate around its axis.

Taijiquan Leg Training on the Ball

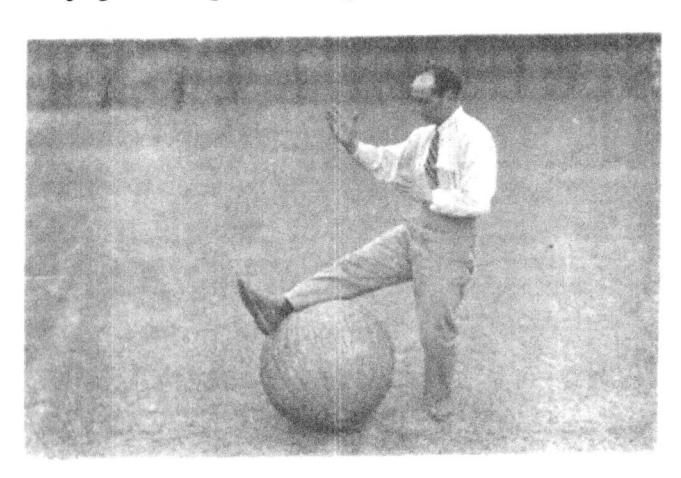

Training the waist and legs in Taijiquan involves using a ball made of bamboo or rattan with a diameter of about two feet. The ball is placed on the ground, and through pushing the ball with the waist and legs, one engages in the exercise.

Fighting Ball Arena

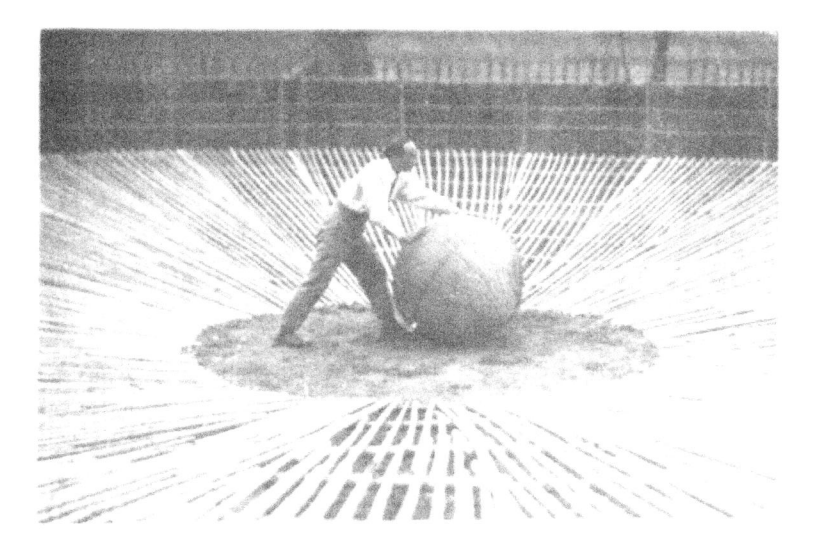

In addition, there is the invention of a combat ball arena. The arena is circular, constructed with bamboo or wood to form a ring resembling a basin. Countless small rods or wooden boards are inclined within it, higher on the outside and flat on the inside. There is a vacant space in the center of the arena, approximately one zhang in diameter, with the circumference measuring two and a half zhang. Thus, the entire diameter of the arena is six zhang. A person stands inside and uses their arms to coil a rattan-made ball with a diameter of three to four chi. When the ball is pushed, it naturally begins to rotate, and its movement is unleashed in accordance with its momentum. The ball spins and rolls towards the edge of the arena, and as it descends, the person catches it with their arms, chest, back, or legs, and then launches it again. In this way, the ball serves as a substitute for a person, performing various combat postures. Once the skills are mastered through practice, when encountering an opponent, one can use a person as the "ball." This type of combat ball requires the use of this arena for individual practice, while for two or three people, or three or four people practicing together, a flat ground is sufficient. As person A pushes the ball, it rotates and is launched to person B, who catches and pushes it to person C. In this manner, when multiple people perform the movements simultaneously, the entire body can be exercised.